To Je

FABULOUSLY FIT
FOREVER
Expanded

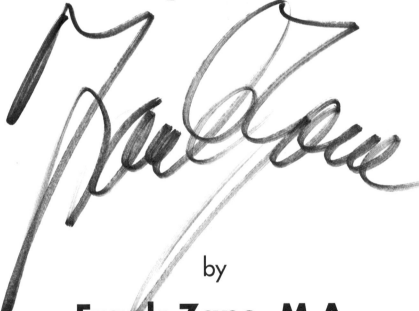

by

Frank Zane, M.A.

3 times Mr. Olympia

with illustrations by Christine Harris Zane

Copyright c 1993 by Zananda, Inc.
PO Box 2031, Palm Springs, Ca. 92263
All rights reserved
including the right of reproduction
in whole or in part in any form.
Manufactured in the United States of America
First Printing March, 1993.
Second Printing March, 1995.

Library of Congress Catalog Card Number: 92-91388
Zane, Frank.
  Fabulously Fit Forever Expanded.

Expanded and Revised 2nd Edition
Includes References
ISBN: 0-9636167-1-4

Cover photo by Bill Dobbins
Back cover photo by Ralph De Haan

CONTENTS

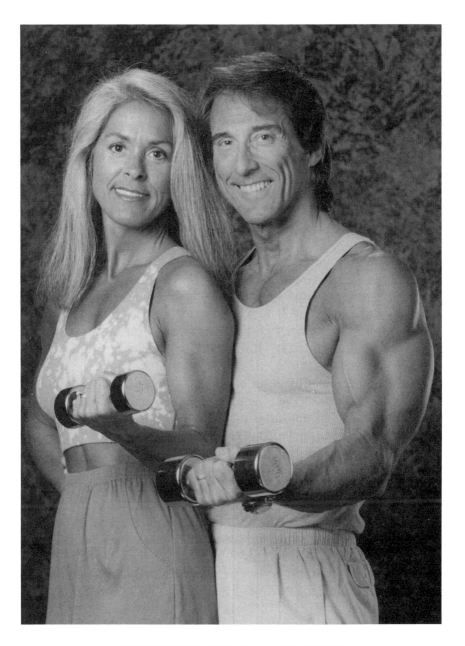

CHRISTINE AND FRANK ZANE

INTRODUCTION:
GROWING YOUNGER

"Our society will become, for the first time in history, not a youthful but a mature society."

Bernice Neugarten (1)

Beginning at birth and continuing throughout our entire lifespan, we are growing, developing, aging. Is it possible to look and feel younger as we grow older? And if the answer is yes, is there an optimum age to begin youthful aging?

Fabulously Fit Forever combines weight-training with aerobics, stretching, nutrition, stress management, deep relaxation, and psychology into a program that will help you improve your physical appearance, health, and well-being no matter what your age. It is a body transformation tool for men and women at all stages of life from youth through "old" age that is aimed at the baby boomers, or people at midlife who form the greatest part of the U.S. population.

The study of developmental psychology teaches us how people's behavior and psychological development change over their lifetimes. Bodybuilding is a behavior which enables people to consciously change their physical development. Integrating bodybuilding with developmental psychology will allow men and women to better understand how fitness directed behavior results in positive psychological and physical change. *Fabulously Fit Forever* is such an endeavor.

Rather than elaborating on fitness at the extremes of age, this book aims at the middle period of one's life. In childhood the attention and intention aren't deliberate enough; in old age, the vitality and metabolism have regressed. Even so, everyone can benefit from regular exercise. Just as some of the arrows aimed at the middle of a target inevitably land outside the center, so will the information I present affect those who are ready for it. The most advanced material is for those most centered.

8

Every year the median age or middle of the population increases by about one year. This makes the percentage of middle aged people in our society greater than ever before. Men and women born during the 1940's through the 1960's comprise one-third of all Americans.

This part of the human lifespan beginning at the half way point is usually accompanied by the realization that our bodies are now less predictable than when we were younger. Middle age motivates us to become more concerned about our health and longevity so we monitor our bodies more closely. We must be more insightful in our training and take precautions to avoid injuries and over-training.

During our teens, twenties, and even thirties we take our bodies for granted. If we have been reasonably healthy and active during our lives, we often assume that our bodies will take care of themselves, hardly giving them a second thought unless we are ill. But as we approach midlife, we begin to notice our bodies are changing. More bodyfat, less lean muscle tissue, loss of strength and stamina, and elevated cholesterol, illness, or injuries often force us to become more concerned about our health and appearance.

This need for body awareness frequently surfaces after a loss in one's life--it may be the temporary loss of health as in a heart attack or other illness or accident, or it may be the loss of a loved one. After such an event people often begin to question how they want to spend the rest of their lives. The realization that one's lifetime is finite brings with it a new sense of urgency for all of us forty plus. Time takes on a new perspective and forces us to wonder about goals and lifestyle of our future years.

People at midlife may have less financial obligation and more leisure time to pay attention to the body. Greater accessibility to modern exercise facilities coupled with a dramatic increase in fitness awareness have made getting and staying in shape the longest measurable American trend ever recorded. But in spite of increased fitness awareness, better exercise facilities and equipment, and more knowledge about the aging process, many people are still confused about how to achieve and maintain the level of fitness they desire. The common sense, step by step approach of this book will help eliminate confusion.

Middle-aged men and women must use every possible method available for physical improvement because they don't have the same metabolism or ability to convert exercise and food into lean muscle as a younger person does. But mature people do have the experience and wisdom that comes with aging. Noticeable physical improvement will begin to occur in middle-aged people quickly with motivated training, intelligent eating, deep relaxation, and a positive attitude. This approach called "wholistic" is elaborated in the pages that follow.

Fabulously Fit Forever is designed to be used by both sexes. Since men and women have the same muscles, the exercises will work equally well for both men as well as women when performed correctly. Don't worry about developing big muscles if you don't want them. A lot of hard and heavy training and eating is needed for muscles to grow large -- it just doesn't happen by accident. Exercise movements done in perfect form along with superior nutrition will insure the kind of physical development you want.

The importance of weight-training as a means to increase bone density, retard osteoporosis, accelerate fat loss, and prevent the wasting of lean muscle mass associated with aging has only been recognized in recent years. In the past, most exercise books about youthful aging have focused on aerobics without much detailed instruction on weight-training. *Fabulously Fit Forever* thoroughly elaborates weight-training and its related areas. My program will provide more fat loss than one that relies on aerobics alone because metabolic rate stays elevated for longer periods following weight-training. This approach is especially attractive to women concerned about keeping off extra pounds as well as men wanting to avoid middle-age spread.

THE BODYBUILDING EQUATION

The word "bodybuilding" means more than building up your body. Bodybuilding really means body transformation. Your progress depends upon how well you practice in each of four areas: exercise, attitude, relaxation, and nutrition. The bodybuilding equation is $B = E \times A \times R \times N$. Bodybuilding success is the product of regular exercise, positive attitude, deep relaxation, and good nutrition. Since the relationship between these four variables is multiplicative, in order to achieve maximum success, you must get perfect scores in each area. Do your absolute best at everything.

The exercise factor is determined by your efficiency at weight training, stretching, and aerobics. This factor measures how hard you train, and is usually given the most attention in people's bodybuilding programs. But by itself, exercise is catabolic--it doesn't build the body, it destroys it. Exercise must be compensated with anabolic factors.

The anabolic factors are rest and nutrition. Rest includes slow wave sleep, REM sleep or dreams, and the relaxation response which you can learn to evoke during the day; together they constitute how well you relax. Nutrition includes macro-nutrition or quantity and quality of protein, fat, and carbohydrates eaten, and micro-nutrition, the amino acids, vitamins, and minerals taken supplementally which insure that you're getting all the essential nutrients you need.

The catabolic factor of exercise must be balanced with the anabolic factors of rest and nutrition. This balance is achieved with right attitude, which is manifested in your thoughts, speech, and behavior and is reflected in the choices you make in your training, eating, and relaxing.

Not only is it important to get a perfect score in all areas of bodybuilding represented by the equation, it is essential to remember to practice to the best of your ability in all four areas of exercise, attitude, relaxation, and nutrition. If you leave out a factor your score becomes zero and so does your progress.

HOW TO USE THIS BOOK

The weight training program you use for your workouts depends more on your current fitness level than your age. The first thing everyone should do is become familiar with the ten stretches described in Chapter 3. These stretches alone make a good workout for anyone who doesn't have access to weight training equipment, but for best results they should be practiced between sets during the weight workout.

Motivated pre-adolescents who have supervision should start with the kid's routine in Chapter 2. Be sure not to let weight training interfere with sports and recreational activities. It's important for children to have variety in exercise in order to develop skills in lots of areas. Elderly people who have never done weight-training should use the program given at the end of Chapter 2 with supervision.

Adolescents and people who have never done bodybuilding before should start with the full body routine in Chapter 3. This is also a good program for anyone with limited time including more advanced trainees desiring maintenance in the off season. If you are in reasonably good shape and have been following a full body training program for several months, you can advance to the split routine in Chapter 4. Or, if you want to lose weight, practice the split routine in Chapter 5.

For those of you who have been training regularly for at least a year, use the 3 way split routine in Chapter 6. This is my favorite way to train and I use this routine when I want to get into top condition. Competitive bodybuilders or those interested in reaching an absolute physical peak can use the advanced bodybuilding routine in Chapter 12.

Pay close attention to the information in Chapter 7 to prevent and treat injuries. Plan your short and long term training goals according to my seasonal approach in Chapter 8. Follow my 4 day eating plan in Chapter 9. Easy to prepare recipes are included along with reduced calorie versions for those interested in losing weight. Practice one or more of the deep relaxation techniques given in Chapter 10 and learn how bodybuilding can enhance your sexuality in Chapter 11. You'll have enough information to stay motivated and train correctly for the rest of your life.

Before you begin training it is imperative to get a physical checkup by a health professional. Do you have any injuries? While it is possible to heal certain injuries through the right kind of therapy and exercise, it is essential to know what kind of training and exercises to avoid.

Fabulously Fit Forever emphasizes bodybuilding at midlife because that's where I happen to be right now in my own life. It also includes bodybuilding in all the stages of life up to midlife based on all the experiences I've had. I must admit that I don't know a lot about old age because I haven't been there yet, but I do know how to extend young adulthood; and that is the goal of this book.

Fabulously Fit Forever is about how to develop the body of your dreams. My intention is to help you become aware of all those areas in your life which are related to making bodybuilding progress. When your goal is to develop a complete body, physically, mentally, emotionally, and spiritually, bodybuilding becomes a vehicle for psychological growth. Not only will I give you detailed instruction on exercises, sets, and reps, but you will also find stories and metaphors throughout the book which describe the human condition and potential. Think about them, question their meaning, and ask "How does this relate to my life?" You may be suprised at what you learn about yourself.

> Secrets live hidden, buried within
> Revealed in words and deeds.
> Dare we recognize how
> They speak to us in dreams?
> Secrets die hidden in body armor.
> Unenlightened inflated ego toiling away life
> Mindless the possibilities of the complete Psyche.
> Secrets lie hidden in words strung together.
> Written and spoken expression
> Mindfully awaken their meaning.

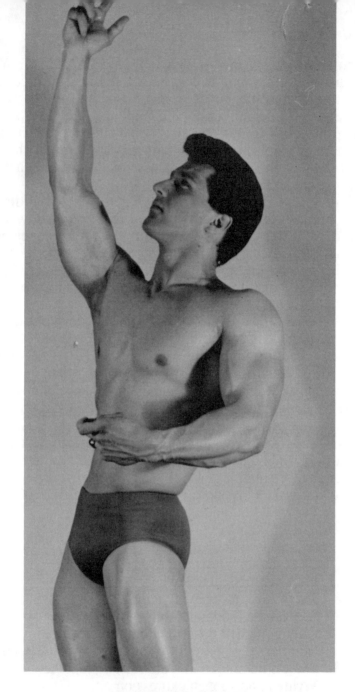

FRANK AT AGE 18

CHAPTER 1
BODYBUILDING
WOMB TO TOMB

"What I am presenting is all against a background of a Universal human experience. We are all born little, and of a specific man and woman. Between birth and today, everyone has accumulated vast experience which we know as the past. In a way, all things you have done up to the present, if you are still around, have worked. The question again is, what is the price and, could the price be lower?"

Virginia Satir (1)

"Everything works if you let it."

Meatloaf (2)

Growing up in Northeastern Pennsylvania, life was anything but simple. As the oldest of two boys, I was shy and had no close friends. My father worked two jobs and when he was home, he said little to me, except when I got into trouble. Constantly seeking his approval, I studied hard and got high grades in school. I spent most of my time in solitary pursuits: building model airplanes, practicing archery, and hiking in the woods. I played baseball, some football, and a little basketball, but team sports just weren't for me. I always felt I could do better on my own.

My father had a good natural physique when he was younger, so it was natural that I was attracted to bodybuilding. Here was a sport I could do myself without having to rely on anyone else. To my surprise and dismay, my father didn't approve. He felt there were more practical ways to build my body like cutting the grass or doing work around the house. Little did I realize at age 14, that I was beginning a lifelong pursuit which would lead to winning all of bodybuilding's top titles. As I grew older, I questioned what motivated me train as hard as I did.

As part of my education, I studied psychology, eventually earning a master's degree. I wanted to learn why I pursued my bodybuilding career with such devotion. What was it in my past that spurred me on to greater bodybuilding achievements? Where did my training incentive come from?

Many of my answers came from Developmental Psychology which studies how people change throughout their lifetimes, and Analytical or Jungian Psychology which delves deep into the unconscious mind and studies its relation to the conscious personality. Its founder, Carl Jung, divided the human lifespan into four parts: childhood, youth, midlife, and old age. Within each of these four stages of life are events and circumstances which motivate a person to begin bodybuilding.

CHILDHOOD

The period between birth and puberty is childhood and is usually the time before a person begins bodybuilding. While I do not feel it is wrong for a child to begin weight-training, it is very important that children are always supervised if they express the desire to train with weights. Since children don't have very long attention spans, their program should be light, short, and simple. Heavy weights should never be lifted! (See Chapter 2 for kid's routine). Children are prone to imitate older family members who train in their presence. Tremendous gains in self-esteem can occur when a child is properly motivated to do a little bodybuilding. Nevertheless, most kids don't get serious about their bodies until adolescence and it's probably better that they are exposed to a wide range of activities and sports that they can have fun doing on their own.

Childhood is an important time in a person's life because this is when personality is molded. One way children shape their personalities is by unconsciously acquiring the characteristics of role models whether they are parents or

16

sports heroes. This process happens through direct or vicarious imitation and is called identification. Object-loss identification, where the child may adopt traits of a parent who is unavailable, is common in childhood. Since boys become masculine by identifying with and modeling their fathers (3), a young boy whose father is missing physically or is emotionally unavailable, may take on characteristics of the father through object-loss identification. In this way, the boy can become more of a man. Although I didn't realize it at the time, this is what was happening with me.

Many of the bodybuilders I know grew up lacking the presence of a male authority figure physically or emotionally available to them. I feel that the drive to develop their bodies is related to a need to identify with male role models. Seeds of bodybuilding may be planted in childhood but lie dormant until adolescence, the most common age for starting bodybuilding.

YOUTH

The youthful period of one's life begins at puberty or adolescence, moves through young adulthood, and continues until midlife. The body reaches physical maturity during this time. The desire to practice bodybuilding usually awakens at puberty or shortly thereafter. Today there is hardly a teenage boy who hasn't lifted weights.

Physiologically, the male adolescent is ready for bodybuilding. Testosterone, or male hormone secretion, starts to rise and secondary male characteristics such as heavier beard growth, deeper voice, increased pubic and chest hair start to show. It is an ideal time to build muscle. There is a natural growth spurt of four inches per year in 12.5 to 14.5 year old boys (4).

Physical development can be further enhanced by weight-training when continued for several years. This muscular growth is often motivated by a desire to overcome a sense of inferiority by armoring the body with a protective layer of muscle. The process of "bodybuilding as character armor" or body armoring begins since it fulfills a need to cover a lack of confidence or feelings of inadequacy. I began bodybuilding at age 14 as a means to build strength to defend myself against neighborhood gangs. As my muscular layer got thicker, my fears got buried deep down inside. I felt safe since no one wanted to fight me because of my beefed up appearance.

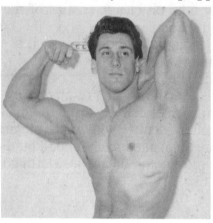

In his book, *Bioenergetics*, Alexander Lowen refers to this process as defensive layering: "The muscular layer is where chronic muscular tensions that support and justify the ego defenses and at the same time protect the person against the underlying layer of suppressed feeling that he dare not express" (5). In this way bodybuilding becomes the ultimate defense mechanism. This is reflected in the many aggressive, violent, war-like metaphors bodybuilders use to describe parts of the body and the training necessary to build them.

I believe there are two kinds of bodybuilding motivation. The first, which occurs during youth, is bodybuilding as character armor. It is motivation out of a sense of deficiency and drives one toward competition. Its purpose is to prove oneself to others and overcome fear, shame and inferiority by building a thick muscular suit of armor. This is synonymous with the development of the youthful ego or identity where a strong outward appearance is expressed and maintained at the expense of suppressed feelings and emotions.

The armoring or defensive layering process of youthful bodybuilding is accompanied by "goal oriented identification" which occurs when a beginner identifies with a successful person in order to feel successful himself. This successful person is the bodybuilding "idol" or role model, and the discovery of the idol is followed by imitation of the idol's behavior, that is, his training program and lifestyle.

We tend to identify with role models who have the same physical characteristics, such as body type or structure, as we have (6). There is a certain amount of "narcissistic identification" involved in the role modeling which takes place in idol acquisition. The following passage from a fan letter I once received is typical: "The one I admire most is Frank Zane. I liked you because of your physique; but then I realized I had your body-type and concluded that I was almost like you." Not only am I flattered by such letters but feel a sense of responsibility and motivation in my ongoing training.

It didn't take me long after I began training to find my bodybuilding idol in Steeve Reeves. Being rather thin myself, 145 pounds at 5 feet 9 inches, I could relate to Reeves' physique because he was proportionate, symmetrical, and not bulky. When Reeves starred in the Hercules movies in 1959 during my senior year in high school, I became inspired to a new level and decided to enter physique competition the following year. At the end of my freshman year of college I won my first bodybuilding trophy at age 18, placing 3rd in the Teenage Mr. America. My competitive career was under way. I began to build my identity as I built my body.

Champion bodybuilders are almost always those who start weight-training in their teens. Motivated by a sense of deficiency, they find bodybuilding to be a way to bridge the gap between their present unacceptable self and their ideal self. Bodybuilding as character armor certainly was my motivation in the beginning and through most of my bodybuilding career. But as my popularity as a bodybuilder started to grow, I received hints about how my ego was getting the best of me. The trophies I won in competition were symbolic of my ego development and by 1969 I had collected over 100 of them.

When I won the Mr. World Competition in Belgium in 1969, the 6 foot 250 pound trophy was so big I couldn't lift it. "My ego was already too big" was the unconscious metaphor that I didn't really understand until much later in my career.

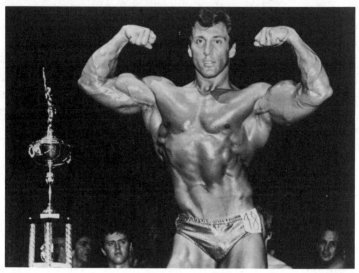

Toward the end of my competition years, awareness of my real purpose in life began to break through my defensive muscular layer into consciousness awareness. There were parts of me that I didn't know. This new awareness led to the realization that I was more than a physical body. The fact that my training needed to progress beyond physical bodybuilding helped me sustain training motivation from another source: Bodybuilding as character completion-- an attitude toward bodybuilding where you practice a more wholistic way of training to grow in all areas of your life. In other words, you train more than just your body. Developing your physique is complemented with training for intellectual, emotional, and spiritual growth as well. In my case, this attitude emerged at midlife along with the realization that I couldn't go on competing against others forever. I needed to change my orientation towards training and start competing with myself to develop my psyche, or total personality, the sum of all my conscious and unconscious psychological processes.

MIDLIFE

"In the rooms where the middle-aged live, quarrels are not between people but deep within the self, and the aggression of youth is turned inward to become the depression of middle age" (7).

Such depression can occur in middle age when a bodybuilder does not let go of character armor and remains fiercely competitive. Driven by conflict and denial of aging, a bodybuilder often continues to bury his inner self by adding layer upon layer of thick dense muscle. I know many such people who remain children trapped inside muscular 40 year old bodies. Still trying to prove themselves to the world, they have ceased to grow in the true sense of the word because they deny their unacknowledged inner feelings.

But while it is true that some bodybuilders never escape from their self imposed prisons, there are those that do. This escape is made possible through the second kind of bodybuilding motivation, bodybuilding as character completion. I first experienced this motivation as a sense of urgency to be in top physical condition yet lived a balanced life. It is synonymous with development of the inner self where one penetrates the armor and gets in touch with true feelings. There is an increase in introversion, reorganization of value systems, and a movement toward self-realization. In the first half of life, ego growth involves the expansion of conscious awareness, whereas in the second half, full development of the inner self implies union of consciousness with the unconscious.

By unconscious, I simply mean that part of my mind, experience, or memory of which I am unaware. My conscious mind is what I am aware of, and this changes from moment to moment. Since I can only think one thought or say one word in a moment, my conscious reality is very limited. The vast portion of the unconscious of which all humanity is unaware is called the collective unconscious.

ARCHETYPES

Searching for my inner self led me through my personal unconscious with glimpses into the collective unconscious. By paying attention to my dreams, I encountered symbolic images of my inner nature, or "archetypes", the prototypes from which life situations are patterned. The purpose and function of archetypes is to educate us about aspects of ourselves we don't know or don't want to know. Repressed from our consciousness or projected on to other people, they live a dream life existence, dwelling beneath the surface of our awareness in the unconscious mind.

Archetypes are like negatives that have to be developed by experience, and although there are many archetypes, the four most important ones involved in self realization at midlife are the persona, the shadow, the anima and the animus (8), and the self. These universal motifs are expressed as characters or symbols in dreams. Archetypes also populate myths, folk tales, and great works of art and literature throughout the world since the beginning of history.

Persona means mask, or the outward appearance a person adopts so others will accept him. My persona was my muscular body mask, my suit of armor, which helped me gain acceptance and recognition in the world of bodybuilding. We spend so much time developing the outward visible appearance as part of ego or identity development in the first half of life that we fail to notice the less obvious aspects of ourselves. But just as the body turns bright when illuminated by the sun, it also casts a shadow.

THE SHADOW

"The shadow is simply the whole unconscious."
Carl Jung (9)

"There is no dark side to the moon, really........
As a matter of fact, it is all dark."
Pink Floyd, lyrics from *Dark Side of the Moon.*

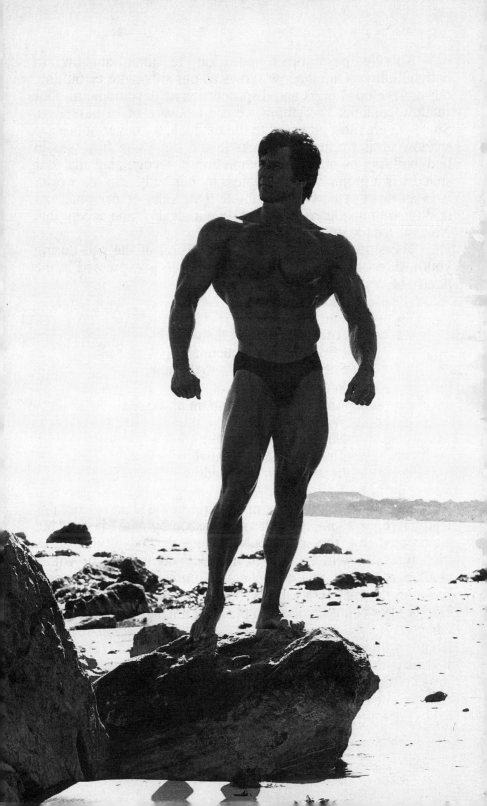

Nobody pays much attention to their shadow in bodybuilding. Our shadow shows us our silhouette or outline, our undeveloped parts and disproportionate development. Our shadow contains everything we are unaware of in ourselves. Since we are most attracted to the obvious, we never notice the shadow until we turn our backs to the sun. The first step in bodybuilding as character completion is recognizing that our shadow is a projection of darkness by our body into the world. It is as much a part of us as our light side, or persona. At midlife we must learn to recognize our shadow and accept that we have a dark side.

The shift in emphasis from expansion of the ego during youth to recognizing the shadow at midlife is expressed in the poetry of Wallace Stevens (10):

> I measure myself
> Against a tall tree
> I find that I am much taller,
> For I reach right up to the sun
> With my eye;
> And I reach to the shore of the sea
> With my ear.
> Nevertheless, I dislike
> The way the ants crawl
> In and out of my shadow.

This powerful, often fearful image of the shadow contains instinctive wisdom, which is sensed by the body, but suppressed by the persona. I experienced my shadow archetype as a wild uncivilized man who confronted me with a challenge. This shadow contains unlived material which becomes destructive when ignored. I became aware of shadow energy after being involved in personal mishaps, as I explain in Chapter 7. As part of my personal growth,I learn to make friends with hostile people whether in dreams or in waking life. I realize that I perceive hostility in people because I often project my own hostile tendancies on them instead of recognizing this feeling as my own.

After shadow confrontation came encounters with my **anima**, or image of the opposite sex, the female aspect of the male psyche. The animus archetype is the masculine side of the female personality. The anima and animus are repressed opposite sex tendencies which have been expelled from the conscious mind. The personal growth process at midlife suggests that men develop their repressed emotional, receptive, intuitive, non-aggressive "female" qualities, while women bring out independent, forceful, self assertive, logical, analytical "masculine" traits which they have repressed.

"Every person has qualities of the opposite sex, not only in the biological sense that man and woman both secrete both male and female sex hormones, but also in a psychological sense of attitudes and feelings...If the personality is to be well adjusted and harmoniously balanced, the feminine side of a man's personality and the masculine side of a woman's personality must be allowed to express themselves in consciousness and behavior. If a man exhibits only masculine traits, his feminine traits remain unconscious, therefore these traits remain undeveloped and primitive. This gives the unconscious a quality of weakness and impressionability. That is why the most virile appearing and virile acting man is often weak and submissive inside. A woman who exhibits excessive femininity in her external life would have the unconscious qualities of stubbornness or willfulness, qualities that are often present in man's outer behavior." (11)

A major task of midlife is assimilating the shadow and anima (animus) into the conscious personality. As part of my dream work process of confronting, befriending and honoring my shadow I was able to channel negative feelings tied up in anger, resentment, fear, shame and hostility into positive energy I could use in my workouts. I also learned to ask my

25

anima for advice and discovered her to be a creative guide through my unconscious wilderness. My anima often appeared in my dreams as a young woman leading me out of prison. This prison was my belief system which forged my muscular armor and kept me incarcerated. Once free, I was able to pursue true personal growth using bodybuilding as a means to this end.

Along this path of self realization, which Jung calls individuation, I encountered symbols of the **self** archetype in my dreams. The self is the inner guiding factor, the organizing principle of the personality. The self archetype becomes evident at midlife after the ego or conscious personality has matured, for the ego must cooperate in receiving messages from the self. Such messages from the inner self help put the puzzle pieces of dreams together. Everyone has this deep inner knowledge; our ultimate goal is to get in touch with it and use it in our daily lives. Mastering disciplines such as meditation, yoga, martial arts, and bodybuilding can lead to a sense of oneness and harmony with the universe.

THE MIDLIFE CRISIS

Sedentary people find other ways of armoring themselves. Rigidity of attitude is expressed in stiffness of movements and poor posture. For non-exercising people who never get trapped inside muscular bodies, midlife is the beginning of over the hill existence and involuntary suffering. Carl Jung referred to it as the beginning of life's decline, "life's noon" and noted a rise in the frequency of mental depressions in men about 40 and somewhat earlier for women. These neurotic disturbances characteristic of the adult years of most people, the midlife crisis, all have one thing in common: they want to carry the psychology of the youthful phase of life over into midlife. "There is a sense of being in the prime of one's life in terms of one's experience and good judgement, and on the other hand the sense of being newly vulnerable" (12).

We don't want to give up our youth and in a sense we don't have to if we take advantage of the benefits bodybuilding has to offer. Bodybuilding at midlife is an opportunity to transform neurosis into an art form. Although it is in young adulthood that peak physical condition is usually reached, the longer and more intelligently one continues to train, the longer peak condition can be extended. Today there are some bodybuilders who are in peak physical condition in their 60's like Bill Pearl, and even in their 70's like Bob Delmontique.

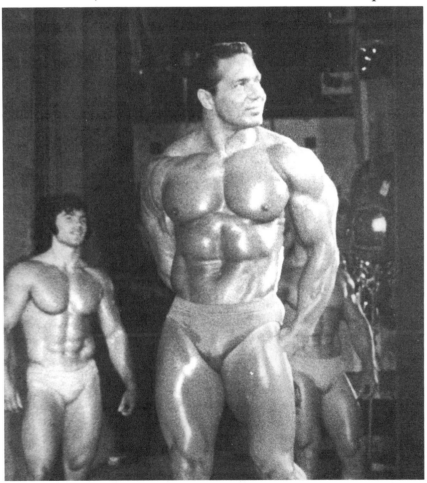

BILL PEARL, AGE 41 IN HIS LAST COMPETITION, 1971

Since signs of aging don't seem to be age-specific, a person can be young or old at any age. Medical research proves that aging slows dramatically in response to proper exercise and nutrition, no matter what your age or present physical condition. Evans and Rosenberg (13) outline a program that controls muscle mass, strength, basal metabolic rate, body fat percentage, aerobic capacity, blood pressure, insulin sensitivity, cholesterol/HDL ratio, bone density, and body temperature regulation. They refer to these determinants of aging as "biomarkers".

Along these lines, Michael Murphy, Co-founder of Esalen Institute, gives evidence of the many beneficial changes in the body produced by exercise: enlarged and strengthened heart muscle, increased cardiac output, lower resting heart rate, increased blood and hemoglobin levels, improved venous blood return, increased maximum oxygen uptake, improved circulation, decreased blood pressure, greater bone mass, decreased degeneration of joints and ligaments, increased muscular strength, improved reaction time, increased ability to utilize fats and carbohydrates, decreased body fat, normalized blood lipid levels, increased mobilization of lactic acid, improved hormonal balance, increased bloodclot-dissolving enzymes and inhibition of platelet aggregation, strengthened immune system, reversal of coronary heart disease, and improved resistance to cancer (14).

If these aren't enough reasons to adopt a regular training program, Murphy goes on to describe the positive mental and emotional results from regular physical exercise: improved academic performance, self-confidence, emotional stability, independence, cognitive functioning, memory, mood, perception, body image, self control, sexual satisfaction, and work efficiency; and decreased alcohol abuse, anger, anxiety, confusion, depression, dysmenorrhea, headaches, hostility, phobias, stress response, psychotic behavior, tension, and work errors. (15). Can you really afford not to exercise?

My years of training have convinced me that bodybuilding is the fastest and best way to change your appearance. Someone who only does aerobics--running for example--will get aerobically fit, lose bodyfat, and strengthen their legs but will not develop the degree of muscular hardness, symmetry, and proportion as a person who practices bodybuilding. A bodybuilder should also do just enough aerobics according to what his/her goals are. Eating the highest quality foods in a way that is easiest and most practical for you along with mentally training your attitude and getting proper rest on a regular basis are the major factors for bodybuilding success. These factors become even more important as you get older.

OLD AGE

> "The memories of a man in his old age
> are the deeds of a man in his prime."
>
> Pink Floyd

As the final stage in one's life, old age is the last opportunity to perfect the art of living. "Who ever succeeded in draining the whole cup with grace?"(16). A bodybuilder can remain vigorous, well-developed, and healthy throughout later years with continued training. Old age might be defined as low ratings in the biomarkers of Evans and Rosenberg. Yet even people with low scores--the frail elderly--can reverse the adverse effects of aging by practicing bodybuilding. Instead of a decay, old age can be a ripening.

How old is old? A lot of relatively young people ask me if they are too old to begin bodybuilding. When they learn they are younger than I am their belief system often begins to change. Old age is more an attitude to be overcome rather than an inevitable physical deterioration. There is only old attitude rather than old age. I prefer to call the experience of advanced years "maturity" or, "seniority".

I've met many people 50 years of age who could pass for my father. They call me "young man" when I talk with them. I am young for 50 because I don't act my age, and they are old because they have gone into agreement with conventional ideas about how a 50 year old is supposed to look and behave. "These are the 50 year olds whose tired point of view and low energy make them seem old, while some 90 year olds are very youthful in spirit and full of life" writes psychologist Ken Dychtwald, whose book *Age Wave* is a wonderful exposition about how to enjoy the gifts of extended years (17).

During seniority there are triumphs gained through survival, which is the recognition that one has had a wide range of experiences and knows about life in ways no younger person can know. The older person has also recovered from physical and psychological pain and as a result can deal with future contingencies. While it is true that there are restrictions that may occur in one's life with advancing years, the mature person can still set goals and reach them.

As age increases, body wisdom increases, but basal metabolism and hormones related to muscle building decrease. There is an abundance of wisdom gained from experience but the body is not as responsive to exercise nor does it recover as fast from vigorous workouts. Still, one can live fully and train regularly during the later years by structuring the environment so that goal enhancing behaviors are rewarded. An authority on enjoying old age, B.F. Skinner expresses this sentiment well:

> "We can profit from a world so designed that we can behave reasonably well in it in spite of our deficiencies. There is nothing new about helpful environments....If you are really enjoying your life in spite of your imperfections you may find yourself to be an authority. People will come to learn your secret and you would be churlish not to divulge it."(18).

Such are the rewards of maturity.

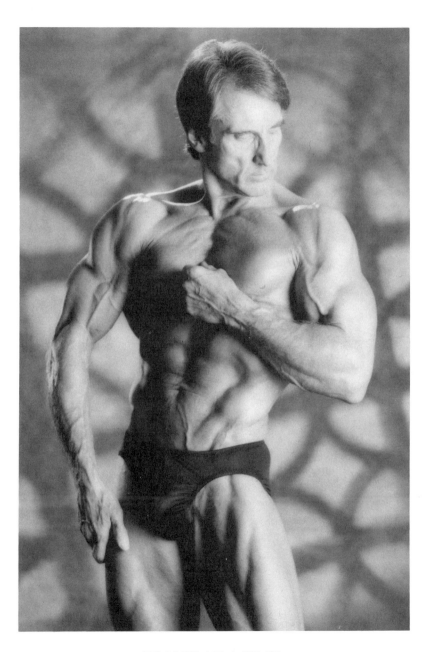

FRANK AT AGE 50

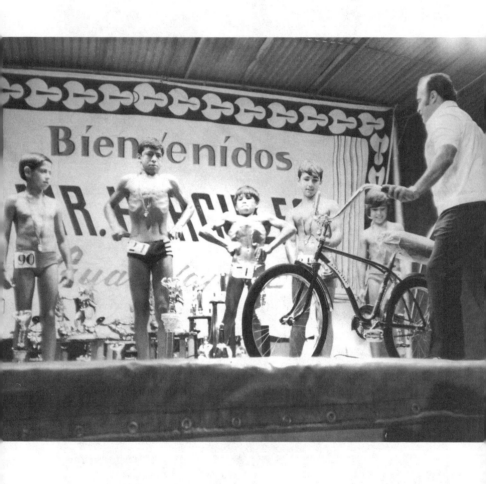

8 YEAR OLD WINNING CHILDREN'S BODYBUILDING
CONTEST, GUADALAJARA, MEXICO.

CHAPTER 2:
BODYBUILDING FOR CHILDREN YOUNG AND OLD

"It is as important for children to grow up fit as it is to grow up smart."

Arnold Schwarzenegger

Although American adults have become more fitness conscious, they have left their children behind. The excitement of outdoor exercise activities must at least match that of indoor video games. So says Arnold Schwarzenegger, 7 times Mr. Olympia and former head of the President's Council of Physical Fitness (1).

Children are the future of our country. It is important that they are given a chance to learn about bodybuilding exercise at an early age. Parents have the best opportunity to encourage their children to lead active lives. Nothing goes further than the example set by parents who make physical fitness an integral part of their lifestyle.

Many people feel that children should not be allowed to lift weights. The fact is that in our society with its abundance of information through the news media, movies, television, magazines, books, and videos, children are usually exposed to weight training at an early age. They deserve the right to be informed about bodybuilding and the correct way to do it and should not be denied the opportunity to train with weights when they express an interest.

The pre-adolescent child should not be forced to exercise. As a former school teacher of 13 years, I learned that kids are more influenced by what you do rather than by what you say. Since I was Mr. Universe teaching school and they liked me as a person, many of my students later took up bodybuilding. Kids make choices unconsciously by two means--identification or reaction formation. They either adopt the behavior of an authority figure or turn against it. How many kids are turned off to piano lessons when forced into taking them? It's the same with exercise. They need role models for an activity that is fun and exciting. Nothing influences children more than being an example in your own life.

Kids need four things to be successful at bodybuilding:

1. An example of a successful bodybuilder who serves as a role model; **2.** The desire to imitate the behavior of the role model, that is, train with weights; **3.** An adequately equipped training setting with proper adult supervision (and participation); and **4.** A system of feedback & reward for getting a good workout.

When the role model, the desire, the setting and supervision, and feedback and reward come together, proceed with children on a very basic barbell and dumbell routine done two or three times a week, where the whole body is worked each session. The workout should be about one half hour long with one or two sets of each exercise. Demonstrate the stretches by going through them before your workout as well as after each set of every weight training exercise. Kids can really benefit from this combination of weight training and stretching.

KID'S FULL BODY ROUTINE

Barbell Clean and Press   Doorway Stretch

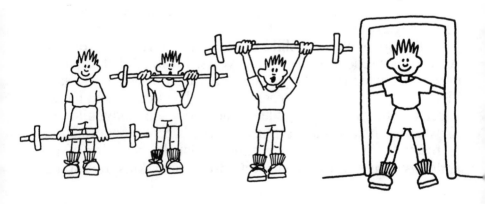

Barbell Bent Forward Row   2 Arm Lat Stretch

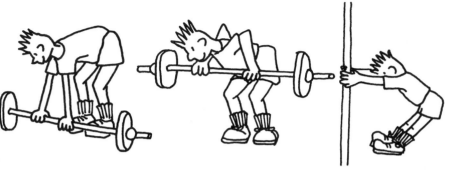

Barbell Bench Press   Doorway Stretch

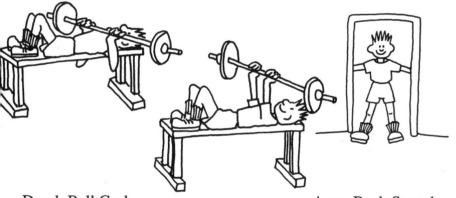

Dumb Bell Curl   Arms Back Stretch

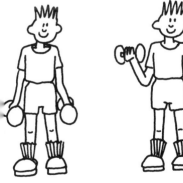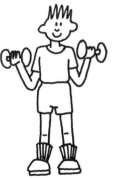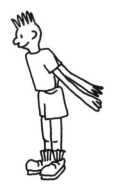

Sit-up

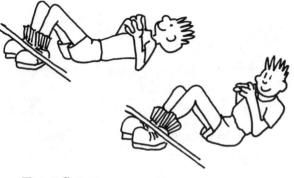

1 Leg Up Stretch

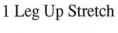

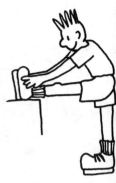

Front Squat

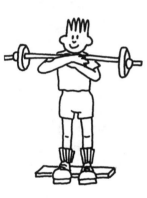

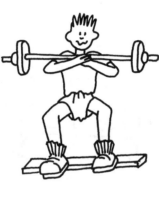

1 Leg Back Stretch

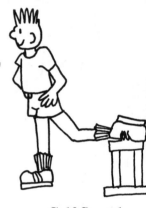

Calf Raise

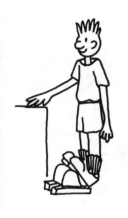

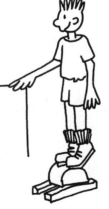

Calf Stretch

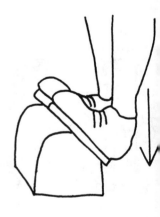

HOW TO PROGRESS: Ten repetitions should be done each set with the emphasis on good form. HEAVY WEIGHTS SHOULD NEVER BE LIFTED FOR LOW REPETITIONS! Avoid exercises like deadlifts and regular squats. Do one set of each exercise for the first month, and when sufficient progress has been made, go to two sets of each exercise. When two sets are used, the weight may be increased 2 & 1/2 pounds on dumb bells and up to 5 pounds on barbell exercises for the second set.

Here's a great reward system I learned from a friend of mine whose child trained with him in their home gym: After the boy finished his workout, the father would stack up all the weight the boy had lifted in a pile. Then the father would emphasize that it took one half hour to lift all this weight. It wasn't lifted all at once and everything was lifted ten times. For example, if the boy lifted 15 pounds for one set of ten reps on all six weight-training exercises, his score was 15 times 6 or 90 pounds, and the father would stack up 9 ten pound plates. If he did two sets, his score was 180 pounds. Be consistent with rewards because kids need concrete examples to be successful at pumping iron.

Kids should also be taught good eating habits so AVOID JUNK FOOD. The best way to do this is not to keep junk food in the house. Candy, pastries, and soft drinks should be replaced with fresh fruit, peanut butter, whole grain cereals, and juices. Again, be an example but don't force them. You don't want them eating junk food on the side. Find alternatives that taste better to them than the junk they've been exposed to. Above all, don't starve your kids --they need ample calories to fuel their high activity level.

A little bodybuilding can go a long way in improving children's self-esteem, confidence, strength, physique, and athletic ability. Do the best you can by continuing your own training and be interested in all exercise activities of your child. And don't worry if your child doesn't stick with bodybuilding. There will be another opportunity at adolescence.

BODYBUILDING FOR SENIORS

"A man is not old as long as he is seeking something."

Jean Rostand

Training programs for senior citizens who haven't done weight-training before have much in common with the training program for children. The main factor is that individuals at the extreme ends of the age spectrum NEED SUPERVISION WHILE EXERCISING. Carl Jung writes "In the first quarter (of life) is childhood, that state in which we are a problem for others but not yet conscious of any problems of our own. Conscious problems fill out the second and third quarters, while in the last, extreme old age, we descend into that condition where, regardless of our state of consciousness, we once more become something of a problem for others."(2)

Since Jung wrote this in 1930, ideas about exercise for the elderly have changed somewhat. You are never too old to exercise. Degenerative changes commonly attributed to aging are actually caused by lack of exercise. Dramatic improvements in muscle tone, strength, and mobility can be achieved through a modest amount of weight-training and stretching.

Studies at the Human Nutrition Center on Aging at Tufts University have proven that the muscles of elderly people are just as responsive to weight training as those of younger people. They observed increases in strength of almost 200% and increases in muscle mass of 15% in the healthy elderly on a weight-training program and increases in strength of as much as 180% and muscle mass increases of up to 12% in the frail elderly from weight training (3).

The difference between children's training and weight-training for the elderly is in the kind of equipment used. Since elderly people are likely to have injuries and are restricted in their movements, coordination, and strength more so than kids, exercise machines are much safer to start with than free weights.

Here is a routine using machines and a minimum amount of free weights for elders that works the whole body and should be practiced three times a week, doing one set of 10 repetitions. Move up to two sets of each exercise after a month or when you feel ready for it. Weight training should make you pleasantly tired and help you sleep better.

SENIOR'S ROUTINE

Leg Extension   1 Leg Back Stretch

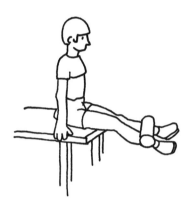 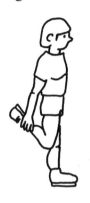

Leg Curl   1 Leg Up Stretch

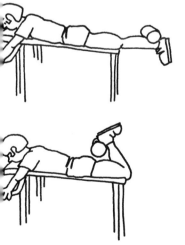 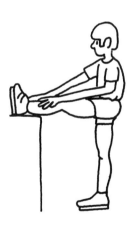

Standing Calf Raise

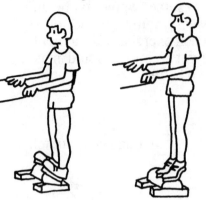
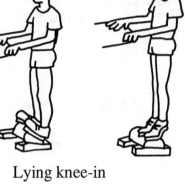

Calf Stretch

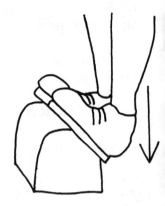

Lying knee-in

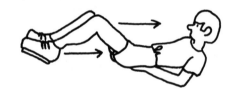

1 Leg Up Stretch

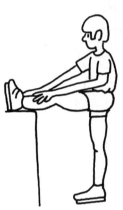

Front Pulldown

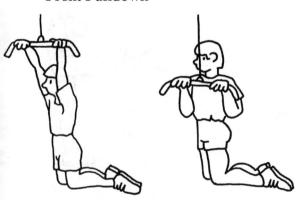

2 Arm Lat Stretch

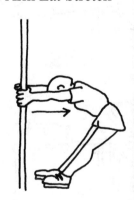

Pec Deck

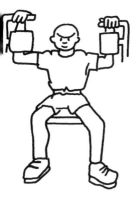 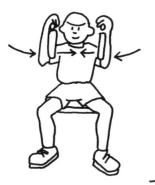

Doorway Stretch

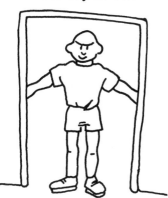

1 Arm Dumb Bell Side Raise

1 Arm Shoulder Stretch

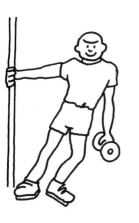 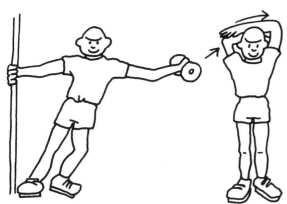

1 Arm Dumb Bell Curl

Pronated Arms Back Stretch

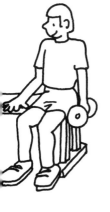 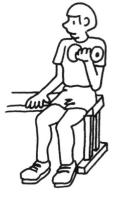 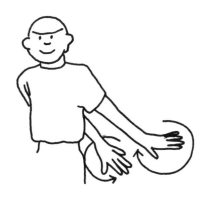

1 Arm Dumb Bell Kickback   Arms Back Stretch

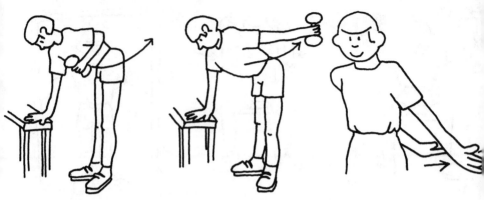

HOW TO PROGRESS: Frail elderly should use the above routine, two or three times a week with light weights for one set of ten reps under the supervision of a qualified personal trainer or physical therapist. For the healthy elderly, barbells and dumb bells may be used exclusively--provided they are light enough-- if you have no access to exercise machines. To this effect, an elderly person can use the Kid's Routine given at the beginning of this chapter, and then progress to the full body routine in Chapter 3 using light dumb bells. After making maximum gains on the full body routine, the senior bodybuilder can begin the two way split routine described in Chapter 4 and follow it for as long as it fulfills one's needs.

The amount of progress an elderly person can make depends upon prior health, injuries, proper motivation and desire to improve, and the right attitude and belief system.
Bob Delmontique at age 72 has made fantastic progress using the three way split described in Chapter 6 because he is healthy and injury free with an extremely positive attitude.

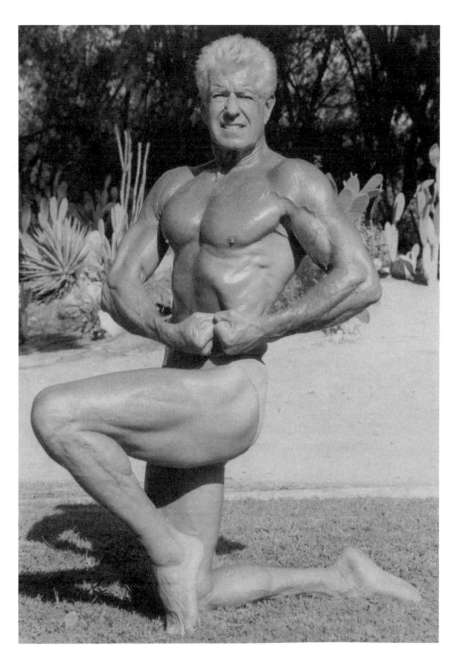

BOB DELMONTIQUE, AGE 72

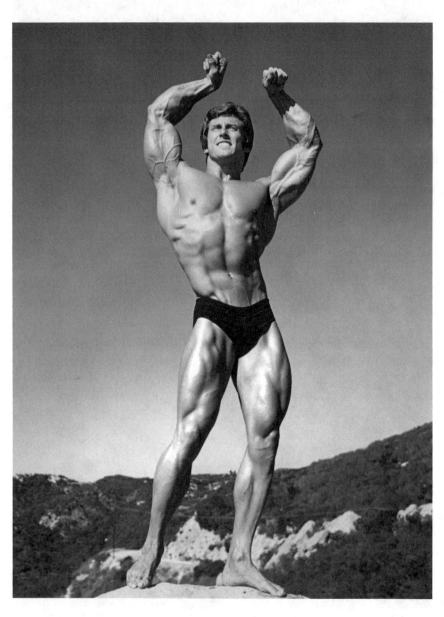

FRANK AT AGE 27

CHAPTER 3
BEGINNING BODYBUILDING

"In the beginner's mind there are many possibilities, but in the expert's there are few."

Shunryu Suzuki (1)

Once upon a time there was a seeker after truth. In his quest for higher learning, the seeker met a Master who gave him a program which would lead to enlightenment. Many years passed, until the seeker was performing his exercises perfectly. People came and watched and then began to copy him because of his skill and success. Eventually the seeker became enlightened, leaving behind him a devoted following of people who continued his way. However, they never did experience enlightenment because they were beginning at the end of the seeker's course of study. (2)

It is important to begin at the beginning! Too many people of all ages who want to get into top condition begin their training by doing too much, too soon. Reading through the pages of *Muscle & Fitness, Flex, Muscle Media 2000, Muscle Mag International, IronMan, Muscle Mag Illustrated,* and *Muscular Development* magazines, they devour the training programs of the bodybuilding champions. Reasoning this is the program that did it for the champs, they'll save time by following it too. Before long they are tired, sore, over-trained, injured, frustrated, and confused. Because they are impatient and not willing to spend time as a beginner, they attempt to complete their penthouse before they erect the basement in the building of their body!

PARSIMONY

The law of parsimony states that simplicity or thrift is necessary when you begin training. Impatience and overenthusiasm can get us into trouble. Why do a lot when a little bit of sensible training is enough to enable the body to respond? Make as much progress from a simple basic program for as long as you possibly can before you go on to a more complex routine. This is true whether you're beginning bodybuilding for the first time or whether you are getting back in shape after a layoff from training.

The more systematic training you've done over the years, the better you can be in the future. The reason for this phenomenon was described by the psychologist Hermann Ebbinghaus as early as 1879 (3). His "method of savings" showed that it takes more time to learn a behavior than to relearn it. Applied to bodybuilding, Ebbinghaus' savings method says that the longer you've been in good shape, the less time it will take you to get into top shape again.

So any regular training you've done before, no matter how long ago, is stored away in your long term memory. Our memory for how to do something, called "procedural" memory, is very resilient and holds up well through old age (4). This prior experience of training will help you relearn faster and get in shape quicker because of savings. Bodybuilders call this muscle memory or neuro-muscular memory.

I remember a time during my junior year in college in 1963 where I became very sick from an antibiotic injection and dropped from a strong healthy 190 pounds to an emaciated 160 pounds. It was a painful experience both physically and emotionally, and I worried about regaining the lost bodyweight I had trained so hard to build. After one month I had recovered from illness and started training again. Two weeks later I had gained 25 muscular pounds thanks to muscle memory! It is like putting money away in a safe deposit box and forgetting you have it. Years later you find the key and discover your money is still there for you to spend, even though it hasn't earned any interest.

Probably the only good thing about being out of shape is that it only takes a little bit of training to show results! My training career has been full of new beginnings. Unexpected circumstances often force me to curtail training for short periods of time, so when this happens, I get back into my training as a beginner. Beginnings occur at all stages of life. But regardless of whether you're starting up or starting over, it is a good idea to begin with a basic weight training routine that works all the muscle groups and combine this with stretching and an aerobics program.

The body thrives on routine! You need a routine to make your training decisions for you, expecially in the beginning. These decisions are what to do, how much to do, and when to do it. The beginning weight training program works the entire body in one session lasting less than an hour and is usually done three times a week on alternate days: Monday, Wednesday, Friday, or Tuesday, Thursday, Saturday. It can even be practiced as little as twice a week for those with very limited time. Since the entire body is worked each session, this program will enable you to improve your symmetry and overall body proportions right from the start.

Symmetry is a balance between the left and right sides of the body. While nature tends to optimize form in the human body through bilateral symmetry, unless we practice the right kind of weight training, we may become less symmetrical as we grow older. The body loses symmetry with age as we continue to move differently with each side of the body. Such is the case with sports we play throughout our lives. Baseball players catch with one hand and throw with another; football players only kick with one leg; tennis players are far from ambidextrous, as are golfers, archers, and basketball players. And while some sports work the whole body in a more balanced fashion than others, such as swimming, sports in general promote asymmetrical development. Through intelligent bodybuilding we can balance a predisposition toward asymmetrical muscular development inherent in practically all athletic endeavors.

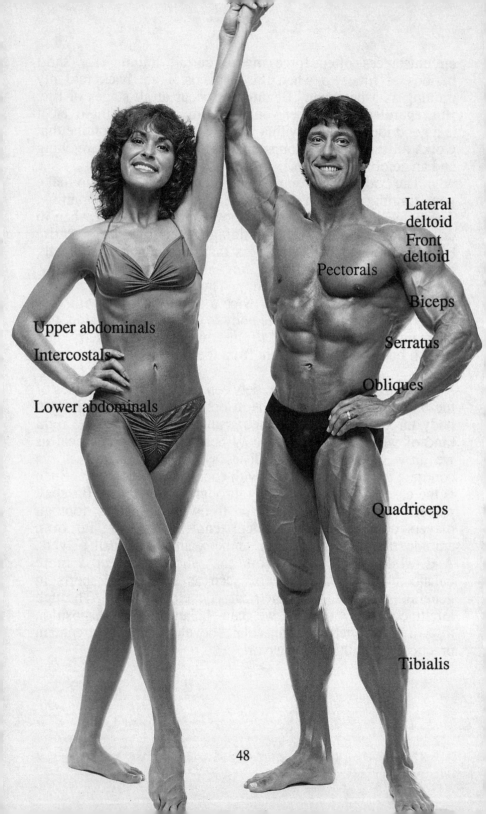

Lateral
deltoid
Front
deltoid

Pectorals

Biceps

Upper abdominals

Serratus

Intercostals

Obliques

Lower abdominals

Quadriceps

Tibialis

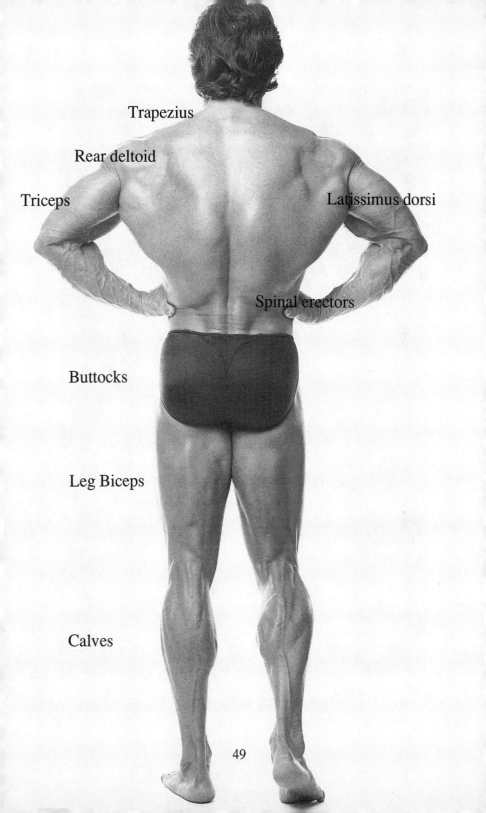

Trapezius

Rear deltoid

Triceps

Latissimus dorsi

Spinal erectors

Buttocks

Leg Biceps

Calves

49

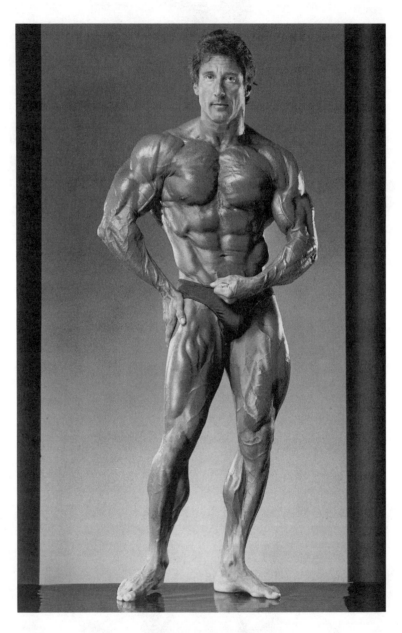

FRANK AT 41, ONE WEEK BEFORE HIS LAST CONTEST

Proportion refers to the overall relationship between the size and degree of development of all bodyparts. Again, sports can create disproportional development: Runners and cyclists develop their legs without upper bodies to match; weight-lifters have big strong traps, thighs, buttocks and lower backs; and gymnasts have great upper bodies at the expense of balanced leg development. In bodybuilding, however, it is possible to develop all parts of the body so that no bodypart dominates visual attention at the expense of the others: thighs must not be too big in comparison with calves, biceps development must match triceps, upper body must not overshadow lower body, upper arms must be in balance with forearms, traps must not be too big for lats, pecs must not be too heavy as to make the deltoids appear too small, neck must not be too big as it would make the shoulders and torso appear narrow, waist should be small enough to accentuate the taper of the torso and development of the legs. Bodybuilders who are considered the best are those who possess near perfect proportion as well as muscular definition, size, and shape.

Muscular definition refers to the degree of development in a muscle. A bodybuilder with great definition is one whose muscles stand out in bold relief. A high degree of definition means that you can see the striations in the muscle fibers. Those lacking such fine detail are called "smooth".

Size refers to how big a muscle is and **shape** refers to a pleasing pattern in the lines of a muscle, such as "diamond calves", "horseshoe" triceps, "washboard" abdominals. In general, muscle size and strength are built by using heavy weights with slow negatives and shape is developed by doing movements in strict form.

A **repetition** is one complete movement of the weight from start to finish (this is called the **positive** phase or concentric part of the movement) and from finish back to starting position (the **negative** or eccentric part of the rep). Repetitions are done consecutively with a smooth, non-jerky rhythm, making sure that the negative part of the rep is always a little slower than the positive. This will give you more control over the weight and help you keep it in the "**groove**" or pathway of optimum resistance to the working muscles. Form should be strict in order to feel the effect of the exercise in the intended muscles. Cheating or loose form with heavier weights brings in other muscle groups and will result in poor muscle shape because the muscles are not isolated properly during the exercise.

A **set** is a series of repetitions done consecutively one after the other. The main effect of doing a set properly is a "**pump**"--a swell feeling in the muscles being worked. It is important to concentrate on the movement of the exercise while counting each repetition silently to yourself, feeling the sensations of expansion as they occur with each rep. The pump will come on toward the end of the set and the muscle will continue to swell in the rest period between sets. You will get the most out of your weight training when you get a pump on each and every set.

Two other factors conducive to getting a good pump are **speed** and **rhythm** of your repetitions. During a workout, your muscles are like a tire with a slow leak. Your negative should always be slower than your positive, but if your reps are too slow and lack rhythm, you lose efficiency and the tire will not get a maximum pump. You stop pumping after a certain number of reps because you get tired and some of the air leaks out which you replenish when you do your set. In this analogy, air swells the tire. In reality, blood swells your muscles. As a result your blood circulatory system develops along with your muscles.

The weight you select should enable you to do only the allocated amount of reps in correct form and no more. Your last rep should not be easy but you should be able to do it in correct form. Do not go to failure--stop before you are forced to stop. Continuing repetitions to failure results in excessive strain on the joints and muscles. Such cheating is an advanced size building technique for bodybuilders preparing for competition and can cause injury if attempted too soon. For most exercises, aim for 10 reps on each set, inhaling on the negative and exhaling on the positive phase of the repetition.

Breathing should be smooth and rhythmic, just like the speed and movement of each repetition. One complete inhalation and exhalation should occur with each repetition, and under no circumstances should you hold your breath during repetitions. So in effect, when you are counting your repetitions you are also counting your breaths. In general, the rule for breathing is to exhale when you need the power to finish the repetition. This is at the end of the positive phase of the rep. People who are in good shape aerobically will probably find themselves less winded after a set than people who do not practice aerobics. They will be able to train with less rest between sets and make more efficient use of workout time which will increase muscular definition.

Stretching (5) is an important part of your workout that will help you make great progress providing you always remember to stretch. The first thing a cat or a dog does after it gets up is stretch for a few seconds. Animals don't need to remind themselves to stretch but people do. Begin your workout with a stretch for the bodypart you are going to start working. Then, immediately after you do each and every set, perform a stretch for the bodypart you are working. Hold each stretch for 15 seconds without bouncing. Stretching between sets like this will help you keep your pump, stay flexible and avoid injuries. Since you must rest between sets, stretching gives you a chance to relax and provides your body with an opportunity to gather strength for the next set. Pace yourself so you complete a set and a stretch every two minutes. We'll use 10 stretches that require little or no equipment:

Doorway Stretch - chest and front deltoids.

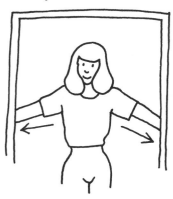
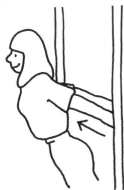

53

One Arm Shoulder Stretch - shoulders, triceps, serratus.

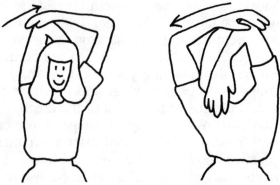

Arms Back Stretch - triceps and rear deltoids.

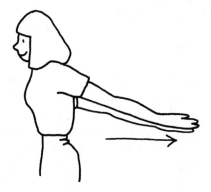

Pronated Arms Back Stretch - lower biceps and forearms.

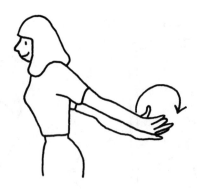

Rear Delt Stretch - rear deltoids, triceps.

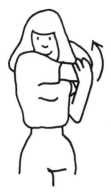

2 Arm Lat Stretch - upper and lower lats.

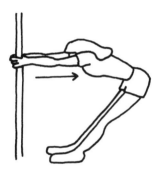

1 Arm Lat Stretch - lower and outer lats.

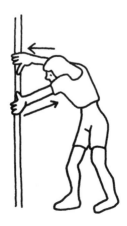

1 Leg Up Stretch - hamstrings, lower back.

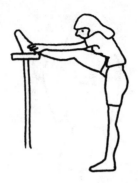

1 Leg Back Stretch - frontal thighs.

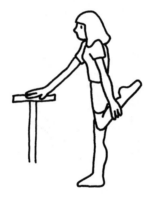

Calf Stretch - calves.

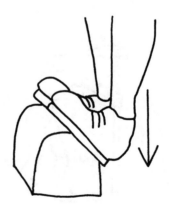

It is a good idea to practice these stretches a few times even before you begin working out with weights. They comprise a complete workout for your entire body and are great to do the day following a workout to ease soreness. The bodyparts you will be training are: back, biceps, forearms, thighs, calves, abdominals, chest, shoulders, and triceps. Aerobic activity is done at the end of the workout. Each workout should be preceded by a light, easily digested meal or snack. Depending on what and how much you eat, you should allow at least 1/2 hour or up to 2 hours for the meal to digest before training.

Getting a good pump depends upon blood sugar levels being elevated enough to give you energy for the first part of your workout. After the first 30 to 45 minutes of weight-training, your body's fueling system changes from glucose to free-fatty acids which find their way into your bloodstream. This process by which fat in and on your body becoming available for energy is called lipolysis--it is the true fat burning part of your workout. Since it occurs toward the end of your training session, this is the best time for aerobics, whose purpose is to burn fat. This is also a good time to do abdominal work since there is little food left in the stomach and ab work involves high repetitions and is aerobic in nature.

Aerobics implies doing repetitive exercise such as walking, running, cycling, climbing, or rowing at less than maximum intensity so that this pace can be continued for an extended length of time. During this time, target heart rate should be reached (= 70% of the difference between 220 and your age) and held for the duration for the exercise. My target rate is 220 minus 50 = 170; 170 times .70 = 119 beats per minute. Aerobics done in this fashion not only burns bodyfat but increases endurance, enabling you to go through your weigh-training workout faster with less rest between sets. Bodybuilders call this "quality training" and practice it to increase the intensity of workouts and get more muscular definition.

57

Here is the beginning program which can be practiced at any stage of life whether you are beginning bodybuilding for the first time (except for children or frail elderly--see Chapter 2) or if you are getting back into shape after a layoff. Since it requires a minimum of equipment, it can be done at home. As a matter of fact, this is the program I first started with at age 14. I purchased a pair of dumb bells that were adjustable from 5 to 15 pounds each in 2 & 1/2 pound increments and began training faithfully in my basement three times a week after school. I was amazed when I saw muscles popping out everywhere after only two weeks! The superior range of movement provided by dumb bells is the best way I know of to develop great shape to all muscles of the upper body.Be sure to do enough aerobics which involve legs, since most of the exercises in this routine are for upper body.

THE FULL BODY ROUTINE

INCLINE DUMB BELL PRESS & doorway stretch

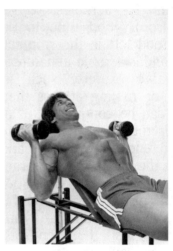 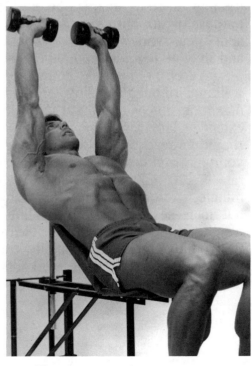

1 ARM DUMB BELL ROW & 1 arm lat stretch

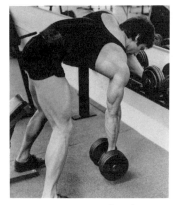 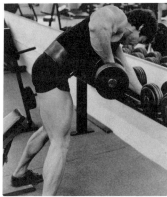

DUMB BELL FLY & doorway stretch

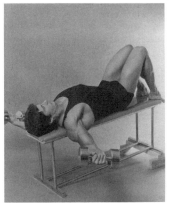 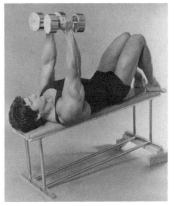

DUMB BELL PULLOVER & 1 arm shoulder stretch

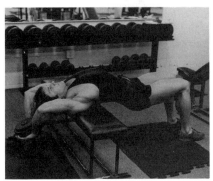 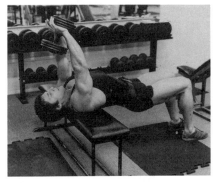

DUMB BELL REAR DELTOID RAISE & rear delt stretch

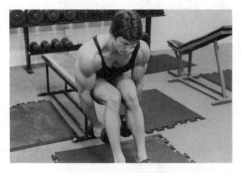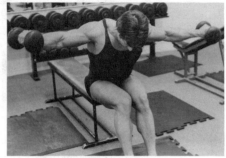

DUMB BELL KICKBACK & arms back stretch

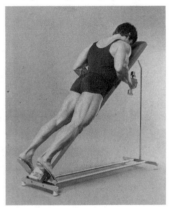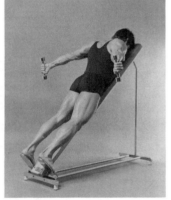

ALTERNATE DB CURL & pronated arms back stretch

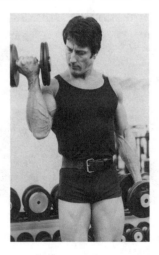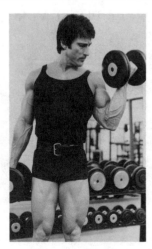

DUMB BELL SIDE RAISE & 1 arm shoulder stretch

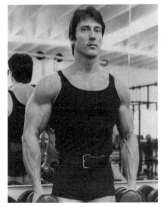 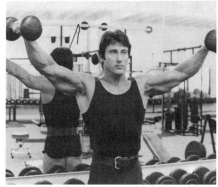

BARBELL REVERSE CURL & pronated arms back stretch

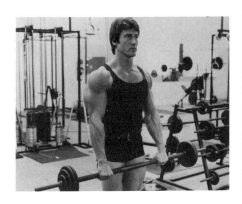 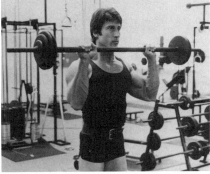

ERECT FRONT SQUAT & 1 leg back stretch

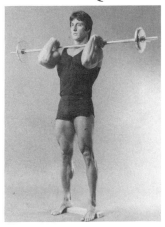 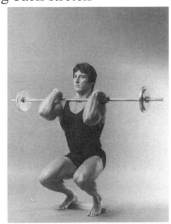

HYPEREXTENSION & 1 leg up stretch

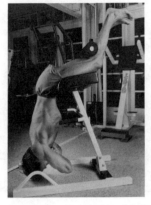 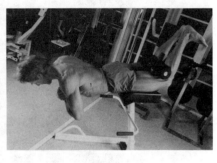

ONE LEGGED CALF RAISE & calf stretch

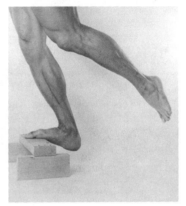 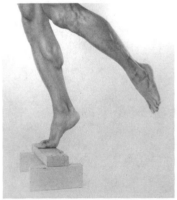

KNEE IN

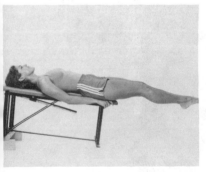 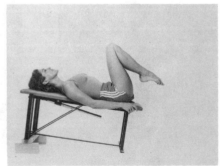

SEATED TWIST

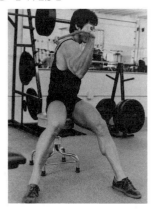 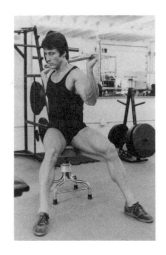

INCLINE PARTIAL SIT-UP.

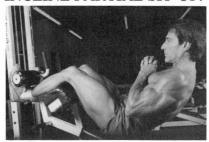 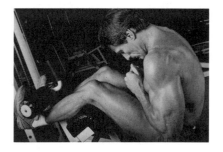

AEROBICS: bicycling, fast walking or jogging for 12 to 20 minutes at target pulse rate.

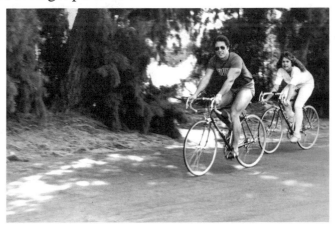

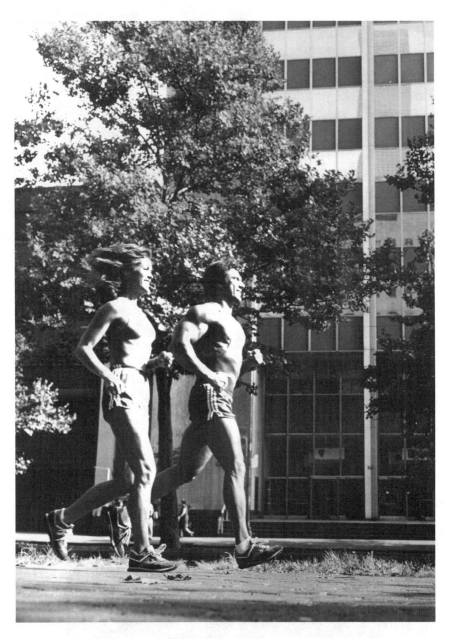

CHRISTINE AND FRANK ENJOY OUTDOOR AEROBICS

EQUIPMENT NEEDED: Barbell, dumb bells, adjustable flat to incline bench, 5 foot wooden pole, squat rack (optional) and calf block. A good way to start building up your dumb bell collection is to have a pair of dumb bells that adjust from 5 to 15 pounds, a pair that adjust from 17.5 to 27.5 pounds and another pair that adjust from 30 to 40 pounds. (Remember you'll need 1 & 1/4 pound plates to make 2 & 1/2 pound weight increments). This makes it possible to go through your workout faster because you will have fewer weight changes to make.

HOW TO PROGRESS - For the first two weeks do one set of 10 to 12 repetitions on everything but calf raise, knee-in, partial sit-up, and seated twist (do 20 to 25 reps on each of these). This should take less than 45 minutes including the 12 minutes of aerobics.

For the next four weeks do 2 sets of each exercise. Do the same amount of reps, but increase the weight on the second set. You'll get a better workout using dumb bells with 2 & 1/2 pound weight increments, since 5 pound increments are often too heavy for shorter rest periods between sets. Do 20 minutes of aerobics. Work on moving through your workout faster by completing a set and a stretch every 90 seconds. You should complete this workout in about one hour.

Now you will be ready for the next phase of training: the split routine.

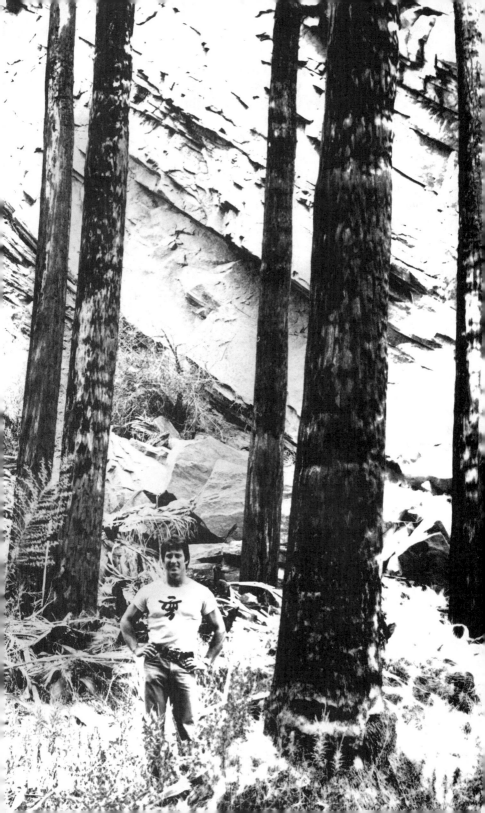

CHAPTER 4
THE SPLIT ROUTINE

Once there was a master craftsman who made such beautiful things out of wood that the king himself demanded to know the secret of his art. "When I am about to make a table" said the craftsman, "I first collect all my energies and bring my mind to absolute quietness. I become oblivious of any reward to be gained or any fame to be acquired. When I am free from the influences of all such outer considerations, I can listen to the inner voice which tells me clearly what I have to do. When my skill is thus concentrated, I take up my ax; I make sure that it is perfectly sharp, that it fits my hand and swings with my arm. Then I enter the forest. I look for the right tree; the tree that is waiting to become my table. And when I find it, I ask, 'What have I for you, and what have you for me?' Then I cut down the tree and set to work. I remember how my masters taught me to bring my skill and my thought into relation with the natural qualities of the wood."

Then the King said, "When the table is finished, it has a magical effect upon me; I cannot treat it as I would any other table. What is the nature of this magic?" "Your Majesty" said the carpenter, "what you call magic comes only from what I have already told you."

Chinese folk tale (1)

"By concentrating our vital energies, quieting our thoughts, and disregarding external rewards, we can realize mastery in everyday work and express our deep nature, or way."

Michael Murphy (2)

With continued practice of the full body routine you will sharpen your training skills. Would this mean that you immediately switch to an advanced routine? No. You stay with the basic routine for as long as you continue to make progress from it. You'll know you are progressing when you feel a little sore the day following the workout.

As you get into better condition, soreness latency quickens. This means that you progress through the soreness cycle faster. If you train too hard in the beginning you may not feel sore the following day, but the next day you may be really sore. When you no longer get sore the following day you need to train more intensely and it is time to advance to the split routine.

The split routine divides the body into sections which you exercise separately during each workout. The simplest split routine is the two-way split where you divide the body in two. Abdominal exercises and aerobics are done every training day at the end of the workout.

This upper body/lower body split is a good routine for anyone who wants to concentrate on their legs, since thighs and calves are worked for one entire workout by themselves. This is a favorite routine of women who want to reduce the hips and thighs because only two bodyparts are worked and there is more time to do more exercises for these areas (see also the weight loss routine in Chapter 5). Extra waistline and aerobic training can be done as well. I like this program because the upper body gets a complete rest on the leg training day, giving it a chance to rest and recuperate.

I made terrific gains on this version of the split routine when I first used it during the summer of 1965 in preparation for the Mr. Universe Contest. Training upper body Monday, Wednesday, and Friday, and legs on Tuesday, Thursday, and Saturday, I used heavy weights: Incline dumb bell presses for 3 sets of 10 reps with 100 pound dumb bells, 3 sets of 10 reps with 325 pounds in the full squat, and my bodyweight shot up from 185 to 205. Since I trained slowly in order to handle the heavier weights, my upper body days took 3 hours and my leg days 1 & 1/2 hours to complete.

The drawback to this program is that there are six bodyparts to train on upper body day, making the amount of work to be done each day uneven. This is not a disadvantage, however, for women or men who need to do more work on hips and thighs since they will be doing extra sets with high reps using lighter weights for the lower body along with more time spent doing aerobics like treadmill, stationary bike, or stairclimber primarily for the legs.

UPPER BODY / LOWER BODY SPLIT ROUTINE
Refer to Chapter 3 for stretches

DAY 1: UPPER BODY

75 DEGREE INCLINE DB PRESS & doorway stretch

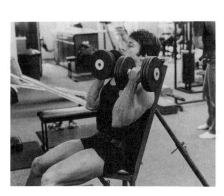
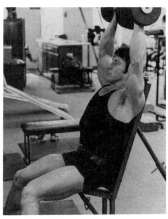

FRONT PULLDOWN & 2 arm lat Stretch

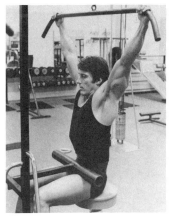
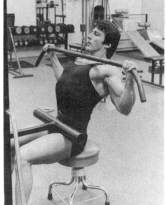

30 DEGREE INCLINE DB PRESS & doorway stretch

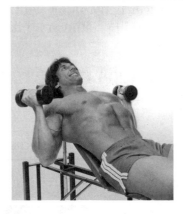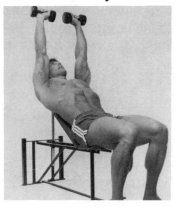

DB REAR DELT RAISE & rear delt stretch

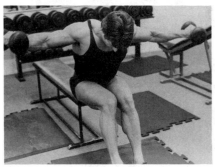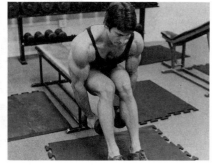

DB FLY & doorway stretch

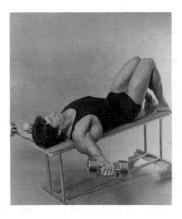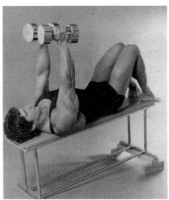

DB PULLOVER & 1 arm shoulder stretch

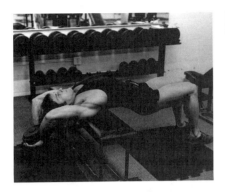
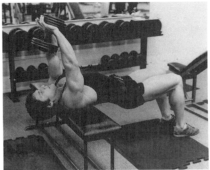

SEATED LOW CABLE ROW & 2 arm lat stretch

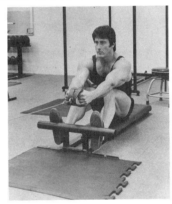
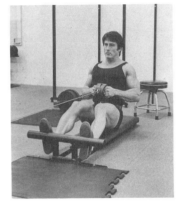

DB KICKBACK & arms back stretch

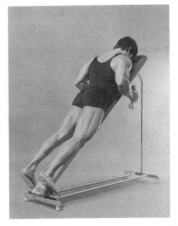
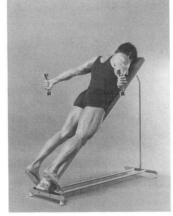

FACE DOWN INCLINE DB CURL & pronated arms back str.

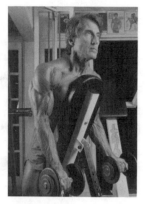 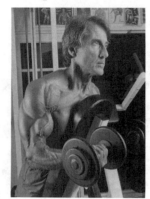

DB SIDE RAISE & 1 arm shoulder stretch

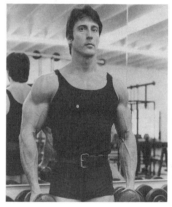 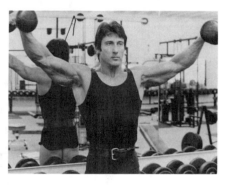

BARBELL REVERSE CURL & pronated arms back stretch

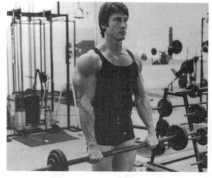 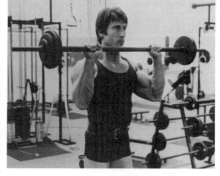

ABDOMINALS:
Knee in

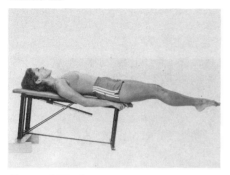 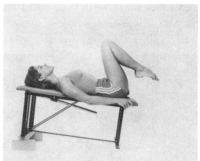

Seated Twist

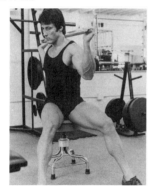 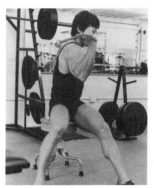

Incline Partial Sit-up

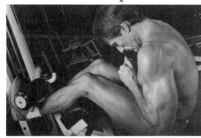 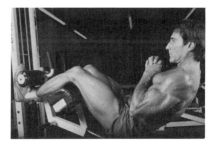

AEROBICS: Rowing ergometer or Airdyne (using arms only) for 12 to 20 minutes at target pulse rate.

DAY 2: LOWER BODY

LEG EXTENSION & one leg back stretch

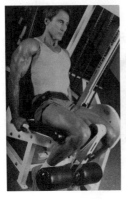
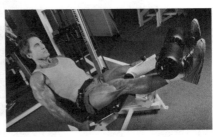

LEG CURL & one leg up stretch

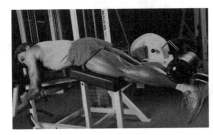
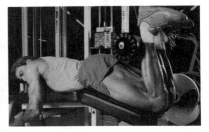

GOOD MORNING EXERCISE & one leg up stretch

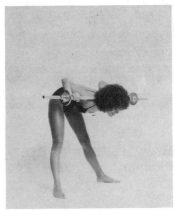

ERECT FRONT SQUAT & one leg back stretch

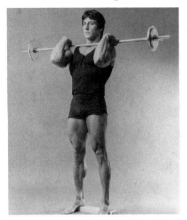 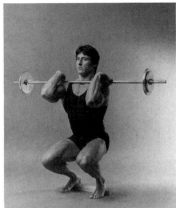

LUNGE & one leg up stretch

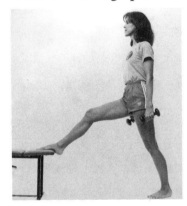 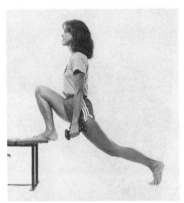

SIDE LEG RAISE WITH ANKLE WEIGHTS

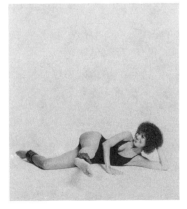 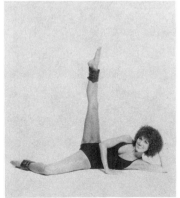

STANDING CALF RAISE & calf stretch

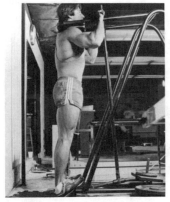 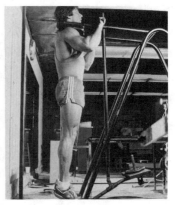

DONKEY CALF RAISE & calf stretch

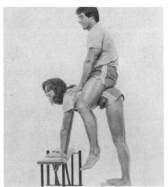 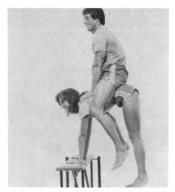

ABDOMINALS:
Leg Raise

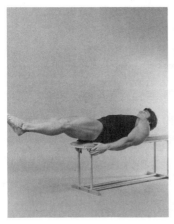 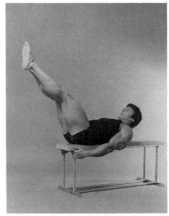

Seated Twist

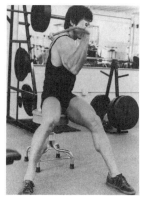 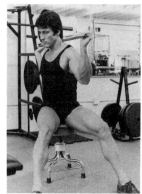

Crunches

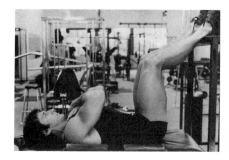 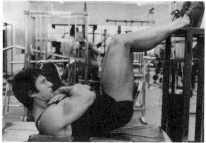

AEROBICS: Treadmill, Stairclimber, or Stationary Bike for 12 to 20 minutes at target heart rate.

EQUIPMENT NEEDED: The upper/lower body split picks up where the beginning routine leaves off because it includes slightly more exercises for each section of the body and uses more advanced equipment. You will need access to the following equipment: Lat machine, low cable row, flat to incline adjustable bench, dumb bells, barbell, 5 foot pole, leg extension, leg curl, Leg Blaster or squat rack, calf block, and ankle weights.

HOW TO PROGRESS: do 2 sets of 10 to 12 reps on the upper body, 2 sets of 12 to 15 reps on the lower body, and 2 sets of 20 to 30 reps on waistline. Do upper body aerobics (rowing or airdyne) for 12 minutes, and lower body aerobics (treadmill, bike, or stairclimber) for 20 minutes. It's a good idea to alternate with a different aerobic exercise each workout for more of a cross-training effect.

To build strength and muscle size, increase the weight on the second set of each exercise. You will not do as many reps on the second set this way and you may find yourself resting a few seconds longer between sets to gather enough strength. To stay lean and hard, use the same weight on your second set as your first set and cut down on the rest interval between sets. This will push you through your workout faster and make your weight-training session more aerobic in nature.

Stay with 2 sets of each exercise for at least 3 or 4 weeks before you go on to 3 sets of each exercise. Remember that your workout becomes one-third longer when you add this third set, so if you're pressed for time you may want to stay at two sets. Many of my clients have been doing two sets of each exercise for quite some time because they must limit their workout to an hour or less. Nevertheless, you can still make great progress on two sets--it all depends on how you do them!

VARIATIONS OF THE TWO WAY SPLIT ROUTINE

The two way split fits a wide variety of lifestyles and time priorities and there are several different ways to perform it. You must train at least 3 to 4 times a week to make this program work for you. Here are some ways to do it, progressing from easiest to most difficult:

3 days a week--Train every other day, or the same 3 days each week (Monday, Wednesday, Friday, or Tuesday, Thursday, Saturday) and do upper body one day and lower body the next day you train.

4 days a week-- Train Upper Body on Monday & Thursday and Lower Body on Tuesday and Friday.

5 days a week-- Women who want to reduce hips and thighs can train Lower Body Monday, Wednesday, and Friday, and Upper Body Tuesday and Thursday. A popular program for building muscle is to train 5 consecutive weekdays and take the weekends off: Monday, Wednesday, Friday -- Upper Body; Tuesday, Thursday -- Lower Body. Then alternate workouts the next week: Monday, Wednesday, Friday -- Lower Body; Tuesday, Thursday -- Upper Body.

Another way of doing the 2 way split is to just keep doing it every other day: Train upper body Monday, rest Tuesday, lower body Wednesday, rest Thursday, upper body Friday, rest Saturday, lower body Sunday, rest Monday, etc. This method is intermediate in difficulty between the 3 day and 4 day a week schedules but you'll need access to a gym every day in the long run because your workout days vary from week to week.

I had great success doing my other favorite version of the two way split: Day 1-- Chest, shoulders, arms, abs, followed the next day by aerobics. Then the next workout was Day 2 -- Back, thighs, calves, and abs, followed by aerobics the next day. I kept alternating Days 1 and 2 with aerobic days and would take a day off whenever I felt like it. I was pleased with the progress I made training this way.

Another version of the 2 way split I've experimented with is Day 1-- Chest, shoulders, triceps, quads and Day 2-- Back, biceps, forearms, hamstrings, and calves. With this version I train only 3 days a week, usually Monday, Wednesday, and Fridays. The only drawback is that if you are squatting heavy your lower back may become stressed from these workouts. You'll avoid this if you squat with your upper body as erect as possible. This program is a prelude to the 3 way split coming up in Chapter 6.

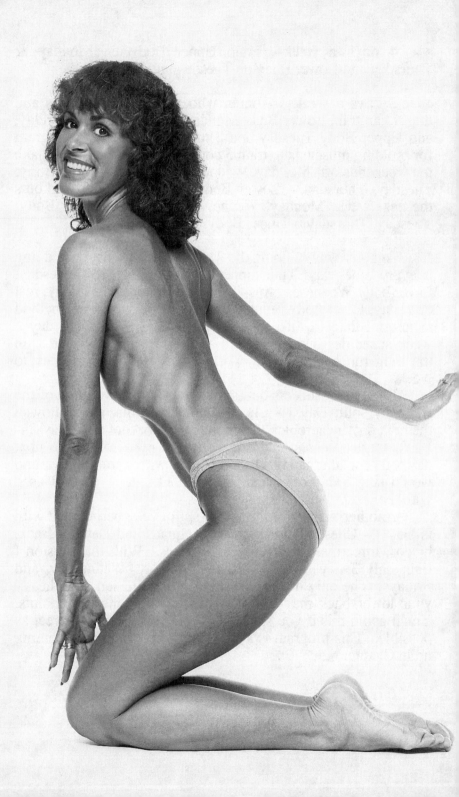

CHAPTER 5
WEIGHT TRAINING
FOR WEIGHT LOSS

Once there was a young woman who lived alone in a land where it was always winter. It was so cold, she put on layer after layer to keep warm, so that she looked like a huge ball. Since she spent all her time trying to keep warm, she was not very happy and felt cold, lonely, and sad.

One day there was a knock on her door from a man who said, "Come with me immediately. This place is being evacuated." But I'm afraid to leave my house", the young woman said to the man. "You must leave here or you will perish" said the man. Fearfully, she agreed and waddled outside as they began a long journey.

At first, the landscape was totally frozen and bleak, but as they continued to walk she began to see shrubs and some of them had leaves, something she had never seen before. She also noticed beads of moisture on her forehead and hands. "What is this wetness running down my body?" she asked. "You are sweating", the man answered. "Take off a layer or two and notice how you feel."

So timidly, the young woman took off a few layers and felt much more comfortable and lighter immediately. She also found she could walk better and saw many new things on the journey: leaves on trees, little animals hopping about, and finally the sun appeared, golden and radiant, and the woman noticed she had more sweat on your brow. She felt so energetic that she began taking off layer after layer after layer.

One day they arrived in a land of shining buildings and beautiful gardens in full bloom with flowers, trees, and lakes everywhere. Catching a glimpse of her reflection, she saw her self emerging from all the layers, slender and beautiful. All around her she saw people like herself who invited her to join their community. And the woman lived happily ever after. (1)

My wife Christine and I have worked with many women over the years and have discovered their basic concern is to lose weight in most cases. True, there are those fortunate women who want to gain weight and this is a piece of cake, or rather a piece of steak, when compared to the discipline it takes to shed bodyfat.

Men and women have different hormonal balances. The prevalence of the male hormone testosterone gives men more upper body strength and muscle and makes the body's center of gravity at the waistline. This is the primary site for fat distribution in men, whereas for women it is located at the hips and upper thighs. Consequently, women tend to store bodyfat here since their center of gravity is lower. Women also have greater hip and thigh strength in proportion to upper body power than men.

I have also seen men who store bodyfat in the same manner as women--flat stomachs with cellulite on the upper outer thighs, and women who store bodyfat like men do--thin thighs with protruding stomachs. Men in this category would do very well by practicing the training program that follows. Women who store bodyfat around the waist should emphasize abdominal exercise and aerobics in their workout (especially rowing which has a more direct effect on the waistline).

Since women generally have a higher percentage of bodyfat than men with more of it stored in the lower body, they may wish to do more aerobics (which rely on high repetition leg work, such as treadmill, stairclimber, stationary bike) than recommended for men. This also applies to men who have excess bodyfat as well. Women who follow this program will probably be surprised at how little weight-training is actually necessary to show progress. A little bodybuilding goes a long way when you do it right.

Here's a program similar to the routine Christine practices on a regular basis that we've found very successful with women or men whose goal is to lose bodyfat. It is a 2-way split routine which should be practiced 3 to 6 times a week depending on how much time and energy you have and what kind of shape you're in. It can be performed with a minimum of equipment or in health studio or home gym.

2 WAY SPLIT ROUTINE FOR WEIGHT LOSS
Refer to Chapter 3 for stretches

DAY 1 - FULL BODY

30 DEGREE INCLINE DB PRESS & doorway stretch

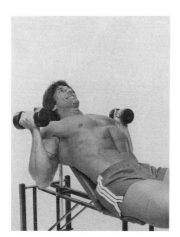 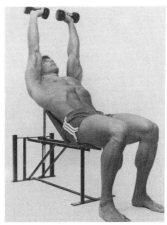

75 DEGREE INCLINE DB PRESS & doorway stretch

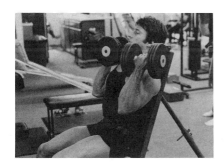 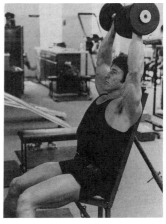

DB FLY & doorway stretch

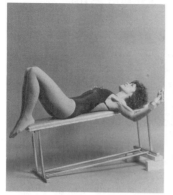 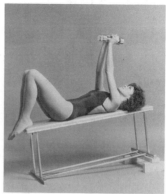

DB PULLOVER & 1 arm shoulder stretch

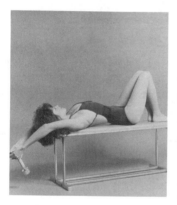 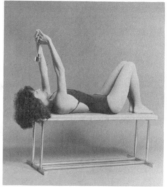

FRONT PULLDOWN & 2 arm lat stretch

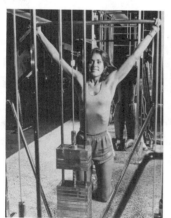 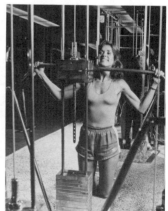

1 ARM DB ROW & 2 arm lat stretch

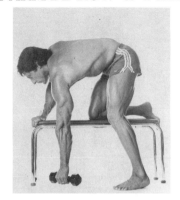 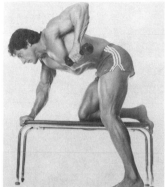

DB KICKBACK & arms back stretch

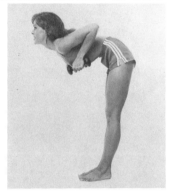 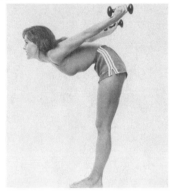

FACE DOWN INCLINE DB CURL & pronated arms back stretch

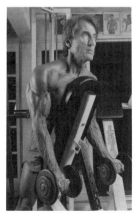 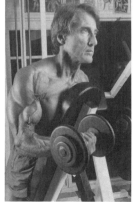

DB SIDE RAISE & rear delt stretch

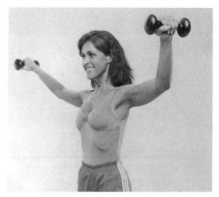 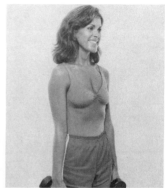

DB REAR DELT RAISE & rear delt stretch

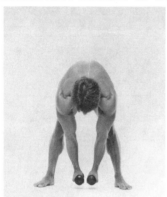 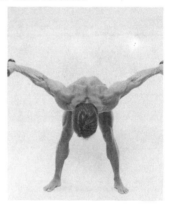

LEG RAISE

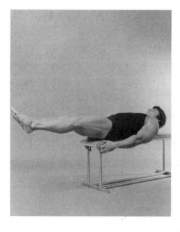 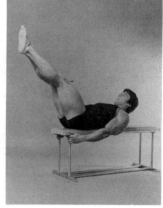

INCLINE PARTIAL SITUP

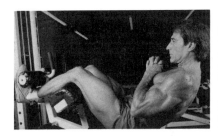 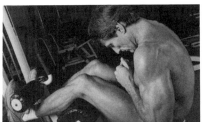

SEATED TWIST

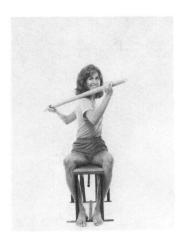

LEG CURL & 1 leg up stretch

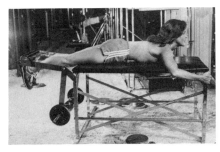 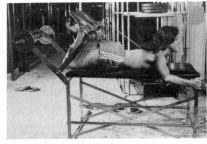

LEG EXTENSION & 1 leg back stretch

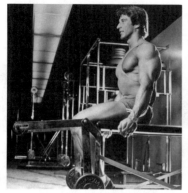 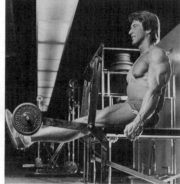

LUNGE & 1 leg up stretch

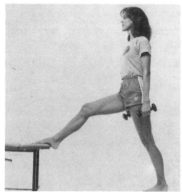 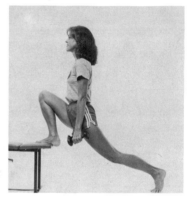

STAIRCLIMBER (10 to 20 min.) & 1 leg back stretch

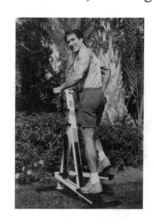

DAY 2 - LOWER BODY

STATIONARY BIKE (5 to 10 minutes) for warm-up

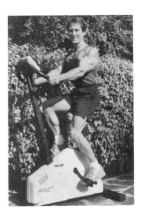

LEG EXTENSION & 1 leg back stretch

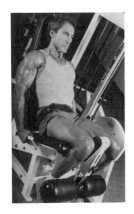
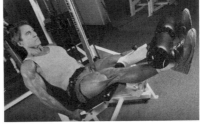

LEG CURL & 1 leg up stretch

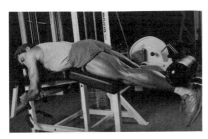
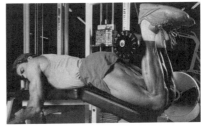

GOOD MORNING EXERCISE & 1 leg up stretch

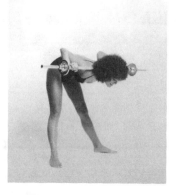

STANDING CALF RAISE & Calf Stretch

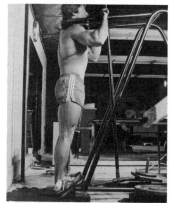 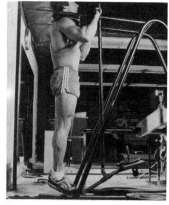

SISSY SQUAT & 1 leg back stretch

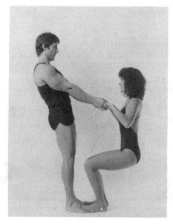

SIDE LEG RAISE, ankle weights, non-stop each leg

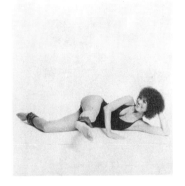 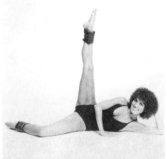

REAR LEG RAISE, ankle weights, non-stop each leg

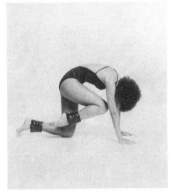 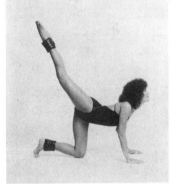

SEATED TWIST

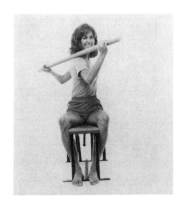

KNEE UPS

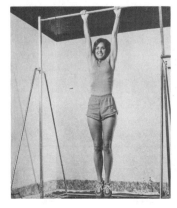 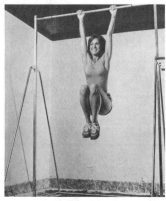

CRUNCHES

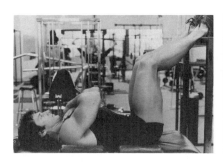 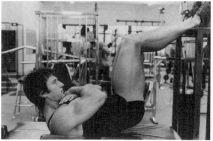

TREADMILL - at least 20 to 30 minutes

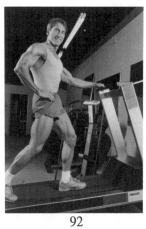

HOW TO PROGRESS: This program emphasizes legs, hips, and waistline since lower body and waist are exercised in each workout. Keep the reps between 15 and 20 and do one set of each exercise on both day 1 and day 2 programs for the first month and then progress to 2 sets of each exercise for the next two months. If your time schedule allows, you can go to 3 sets of each exercise thereafter. In any case, don't do more than you need to. If you are getting sore from the level you are at, stay there until you cease to make progress. And remember the parsimony principle--make the most progress form the least amount of time spent in the gym by concentrating on doing everything correctly.

Keep the pace fast, completing a set and a stretch every two minutes or less. This program can be done alternating every other day: Day 1 on Monday, Day 2 on Wednesday, Day 1 Friday, Day 2 Monday, etc. This is a good way to start for the first two weeks. Then for quicker results and after the soreness subsides a little, do the program 4 days a week: Day 1 on Mondays and Thursdays, Day 2 on Tuesdays and Fridays. Or if you are reasonably fit, have the time and the energy, and want fast results you can do it 5 or 6 days a week by alternating Day 1 and Day 2 on successive days.

Keeping a fast pace in the workout makes your training more aerobic in nature. Forget about lifting heavy weights. concentrate on high reps in perfect form instead. Always finish up your workout with aerobic work which is approximately as long as your weight-training workout, or eventually even longer. Treadmill, stairclimber, airdyne, and Nordic Skier burn the most calories--up to 12 calories per minute-- so be sure to include at least one of these activities every workout. If you are really enthusiastic and are willing to train twice a day, you can make even faster progress. In this case do aerobics separately. You might train with weights in the morning and do aerobics in the late afternoon. This activates your metabolism twice a day and you will burn more calories, so be sure to get enough rest if you train this way.

AB-AEROBICS is a system for losing inches from the waistline and developing cardio-vascular fitness that combines aerobics with abdominal work. Since you need to do both aerobics as well as abdominal work, it is a great time saver to do them simultaneously by practicing ab-aerobics. This system is a form of circuit training where you go from one station to the next, exercising for 45 seconds to one minute at each station. You can work your whole body this way and get an aerobic effect with concentration on the waistline in only 20 minutes. Simply arrange what stationary aerobic equipment you have with your abdominal exercises. The more equipment you have, the bigger the circuit and therefore more people can train together at the same time. Here's a beginning program where you spend 45 seconds on each station plus 15 seconds to change, allowing you to go through the circuit in six minutes:

LEG RAISE STATIONARY BIKE

ROWING MACHINE CRUNCHES

SEATED TWIST STAIRCLIMBER

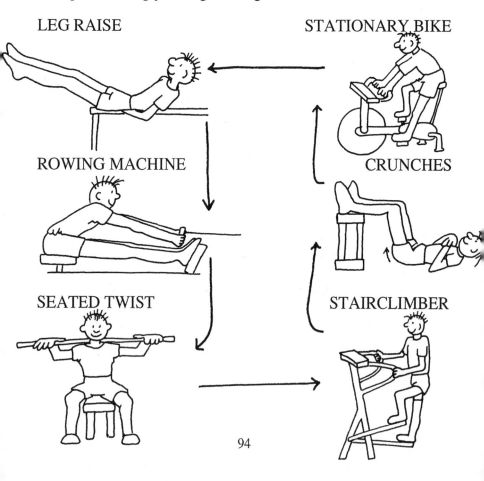

Notice that exercises are arranged so that a stationary aerobic device comes between the abdominal exercises. As you get stronger with more endurance on this program, you can work up to one minute on each station and go around twice. This would enable you to get a great ab-aerobic workout in about 15 minutes.

Here is the ab-aerobic circuit we have permanently installed around the perimeter of our gym:

ADVANCED AB-AEROBIC CIRCUIT

INCLINE KNEE UP	for lower abs, upper thighs
ROWING MACHINE	aerobics,back,waistline,arms
INCLINE PARTIAL SITUP	upper abdominals
STATIONARY BIKE	aerobics, quadriceps, calves
FLAT LEG RAISE	lower abs, frontal upper thighs
STAIRCLIMBER	aerobics, thighs, hips, calves
HYPEREXTENSION	lowerback,buttocks,leg biceps
TREADMILL	aerobics, thighs, hips, calves
SEATED TWIST	obliques, stretches lower back
CRUNCHES	upper abdominals
AIRDYNE	aerobics, upper body, legs

Technically speaking, an exercise like rowing or stationary bike is not aerobic unless it is done for a minimum of 12 minutes at target heart rate. The overall effect of these exercises, however, is aerobic because the heart rate stays elevated for as long as you do the circuit, which should be at least 12 minutes.

Some good advice is not to put two abdominal exercises next to each other that work the same area, like crunches following partial sit-up (both work upper abs), or incline knee ups following leg raise (both work lower abs). This is a program which can be done all the time as your regular aerobic plus abdominal routine or you can use it for group classes with friends.

AEROBICS

Another way to train abdominals and aerobics is to do them separately. For best results, do this training at the end of your weight-training program, or in another training session the same day. Here are some of our favorite forms of aerobics:

Rowing - 500 to 2500 meters (4 to 15 minutes) after upper body work at a cadence of 25 to 35 strokes per minute.

Stairclimber - 12 or more minutes at a rapid pace taking short steps and easy resistance.

Stationary Bike - 12 to 30 minutes at a cadence of 90 revolutions per minute after leg workout.

Treadmill - Can be done at a separate time for 20 to 45 minutes walking at 3 to 4 miles per hour for prolonged caloric expenditure. Of course you can walk outside without a treadmill.

Airdyne - 12 to 30 minutes at the end of your leg or upper body workouts works your whole body and burns a lot of calories.

Aerobic dance or step classes are a good way to get your aerobic activity in by taking advantage of a group and a leader. They are also less boring for most people.

AEROBICS OR AB-AEROBICS?

Some criteria for deciding whether to do ab-aerobics or abdominals and aerobics separately are:

1. Ab-aerobics are great for small groups of people. you can experience a tremendous "group spirt" or motivating force by feeding off each other's energy.

2. you may wish to do your aerobic exercise outdoors if the weather is nice. If so, I recommend fast walking as the most pleasurable and safest outdoor aerobic activity.

3. If you are training alone or with a partner and you must do all your exercise in the gym, you can use either method. Ab-aerobics is difficult to do in a commercial gym because you need many pieces of equipment which other people are using, so you might separate ab work from aerobics in this case due equipment availability.

It is also very important not to eat much after 5 or 6 pm. Follow the restricted calorie version of the eating plan in Chapter 9 and never eat starches late in the day. The restricted calorie version reduces portion sizes, making the diet lower in calories. Keep your fat intake under 20% of your total calories, and stay under 8 calories per pound of desired bodyweight. Stick to this program no matter how long it takes and you will be rewarded for your efforts. Gradual weight loss averaging one pound a week or slightly more is safest and will give more lasting results. Ask yourself how long it took you to gain the weight you now want to lose. You can't be in a hurry and expect to lose weight safely.

ATTITUDE TOWARD EATING AND EXERCISE

Your self-concept has much to do with success or failure on a weight loss program. For best results, do everything possible to maintain a positive attitude. This includes what you think about yourself and how you express it in your speech. The statement "I am 15 pounds overweight" has a different self-conception when associated with "I could be quite thin" rather than "I will always be fat"(2). Every day visualize the possible self you want to become (use the Dream Body Visualization in Chapter 12) and make this your incentive for the behavior necessary to achieve your weight loss goals.

Christine and I have noticed a positive correlation between our individual bodyweights and the shape we're in. When she is training hard and in great shape so am I. Our relationship of over 25 years has enabled us to share the same goals and values and this is expressed in our training behavior. We realize how we influence each other by our attitudes toward training.

Christine was my training partner for the 1979 Mr. Olympia. Some people at the gym thought I would never get into top condition, but I got into the best shape of my life that year and so did she. Right company is very important when you want to be and do your very best. By associating with people who have similar goals, you will grow in a positive way, so maximize your environment!

In the words of Wallace Stevens (3):

> I am what is around me.
> Women understand this.
> One is not a duchess
> A hundred yards from a carriage.

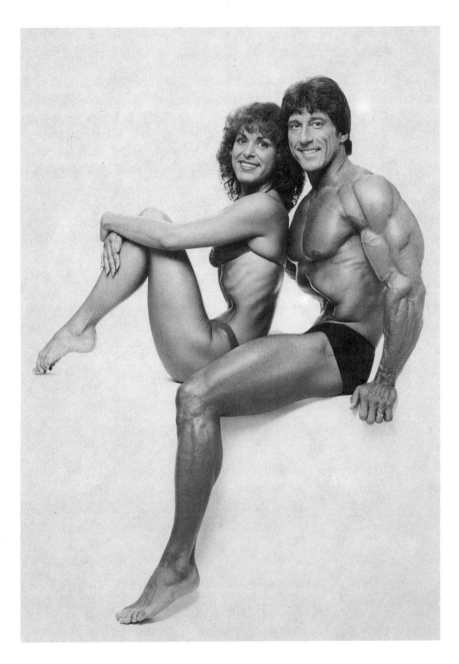

CHRISTINE & FRANK 1979, AFTER 3RD OLYMPIA WIN

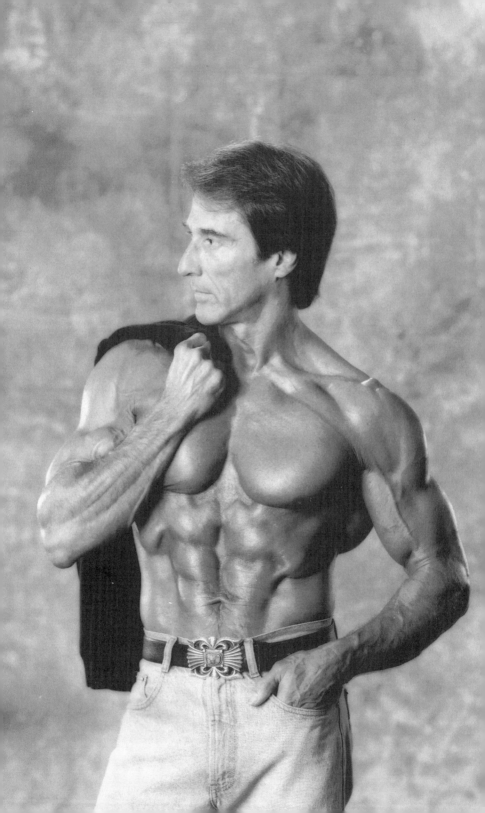

CHAPTER 6
THE 3 WAY
SPLIT ROUTINE

Man as a whole is comparable to a carriage, a horse, and a coachman...The difference between a real man and a pseudo man is indicated by the passenger in the carriage. In the case of the real man, the passenger is the owner of the carriage; and in the pseudo man, he is simply the first chance passer-by who, like the fare in a hackney carriage, is continuously being changed.

The body of a man with all its motor reflexes corresponds to the carriage itself; all the functionings and manifestations of feeling of a man correspond to the horse harnessed to the carriage and drawing it; the coachman sitting on the carriage and directing the horse corresponds to a man's consciousness (or mind); and finally, the passenger seated in the carriage and commanding the coachman is that which is called "I" (or inner self).

This "I", which should be present in everybody on reaching responsible age, is entirely missing in them. Almost every contemporary man consists of a broken down carriage which has long ago seen its day, a crock of a horse, and a half-drunken coachman whose time designated by Mother Nature for self-perfection passes while he waits on a corner, fantastically daydreaming, for any chance passenger.

Every man should strive to have his own "I"; otherwise he will always represent a hackney carriage in which any fare can sit and which any fare can dispose of as he pleases.(1)

To make real progress in bodybuilding, you must master a variety of exercises by learning to perform them perfectly. There is no better way to do this than with the three way split routine. This program divides the body into three segments so you can concentrate more deeply and do more work for each bodypart and allow more time to progress through the soreness cycle. One of the problems with a full body workout, or even an upper body workout, is that there are too many bodyparts to work in one session. Your attention span and energy fade as your workout lengthens so what gets worked last usually gets worked least.

Since you never work more than three bodyparts plus abdominals in one session, your training motivation will be better for each workout. Organizing your program in this way will enable you to develop great shape and proportion to all your muscles.

Although there are different ways to split up the body, the method that makes the most sense is to split according to function, that is, train muscles that work the same way during the same workout. My favorite way is:

Day 1 - Pulling muscles: Back, biceps, forearms.
Day 2 - Leg muscles: Thighs, calves.
Day 3 - Pushing muscles: Chest, shoulders, triceps.
Abdominal work is done every training day along with aerobics at the end of your workout.

Day 1 and day 3 can be interchanged but Day 2, Legs, must always be done between days 1 and 3 in order to give the upper body adequate time to rest. Certain parts of the upper body such as shoulders and elbows are worked on every upper body exercise that you do. I know bodybuilders who have chronic shoulder and/or elbow pain because in reality they are stressing these areas every day. For example, if you train back, biceps, forearms on day 1, shoulders and legs on day 2, and chest and triceps on day 3, you are really working shoulders and elbows every day, allowing them no time to recuperate and heal. See Chapter 8 for how often to do these workouts.

A precaution the mature bodybuilder must take is to avoid stressing the joints and vulnerable areas: shoulders, elbows, knees, and lower back. Adequate rest between workouts, proper warm-up and stretching, and keeping these areas warm during the workout are the best preventive measures. Avoiding injury is essential for training longevity. However, I know few bodybuilders who do not have injuries, especially the older ones. Remember, once you get an injury it tends to remain with you for life, either chronically or in latent form, ready to recur at the slightest provocation. I can give you good advice about this because I've incurred my share of injuries over the years. Hopefully I can pass along what I've learned and save you some grief. But more about this in Chapter 7.

THE 3 WAY SPLIT ROUTINE
Refer to Chapter 3 for stretches

DAY 1 - BACK, BICEPS, FOREARMS

Back
>   FRONT PULLDOWN & 2 arm lat stretch
>   SEATED LOW CABLE ROW & 2 arm lat stretch
>   BENT OVER DB UPRIGHT ROW & 2 arm lat stretch
>   ONE ARM DB ROW & 1 arm lat stretch

Biceps
>   ALTERNATE DB CURL & pronated arms back stretch
>   FACE DOWN INCLINE DB CURL & same stretch
>   INCLINE DB CURL & same stretch

Forearms
>   BB REVERSE CURL & pronated arms back stretch
>   BARBELL WRIST CURL & same stretch

In addition to working the entire back, this program works the shoulders as well, especially the rear deltoids. Since pulling movements are used to work the back, biceps are directly involved as well as forearms. Front deltoids are also worked on curling movements and triceps get activated slightly at the completion of the positive phase on pulling movements. Thus the entire body gets worked directly or indirectly.

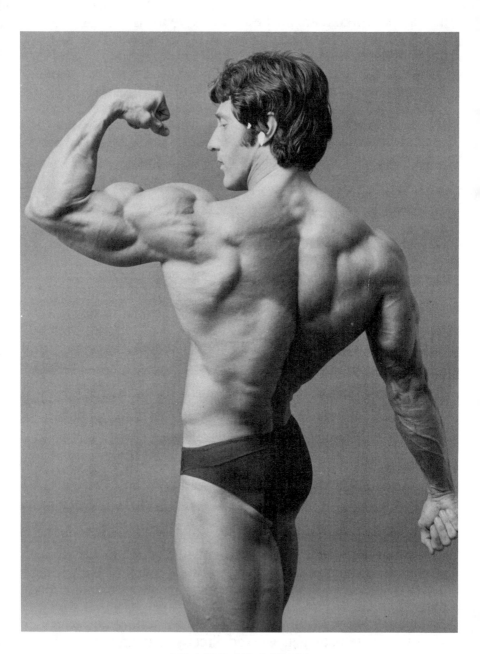

FRANK AT AGE 34

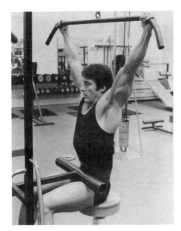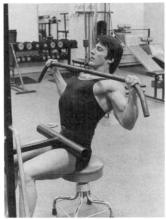

Front pulldown works the upper lats. Be sure to pull the bar all the way down to the upper chest as you lean slightly backward and, without pausing, return the bar until the elbows are slightly bent.

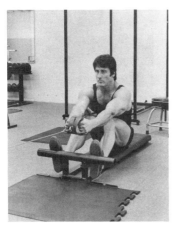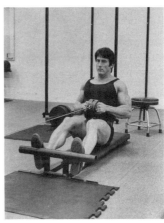

Seated low cable row hits the lower central lats. Pull the handles to the ribcabe, arch the back slightly, and without pausing, return the handles slowly until the elbows are slightly bent, reaching slightly forward as you do so. Be sure to keep the knees bent to avoid stressing the lower back.

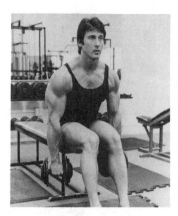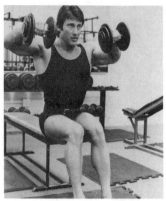

Bent over DB upright row gets the trapezius area between the shoulder blades. Pull the DBs upward until they touch the front deltoids and then lower slowly until they are in line with your hips.

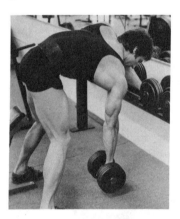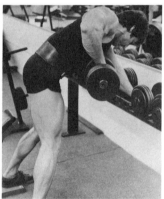

1 arm DB row develops the outer lower lat. Be sure to keep the knees bent to minimize lower back strain and pull the DB up until it touches right under the pectoral, and without pausing, lower the DB all the way down until it almost touches the floor.

"Lat" is short for latissimus dorsi which means "widest muscle" in Latin. Although this back routine emphasizes developing width to the lats, it works all the other muscle groups in the back as well: trapezius, teres major and minor, infraspinatus, superspinatus, rhomboids, and spinal erectors.

I have always taken special precautions to avoid developing the trapezius too thick, so I have not included exercises like shrugs, power cleans, deadlifts, and barbell upright row. These exercises build vertical height to the traps which if overdone will make the shoulders and lats appear narrow. They will also develop the neck and build thickness to the upper back (and spinal erectors in the case of deadlifts). I'm not saying this is bad--it all depends upon what type of look you want for your upper body. I've always preferred width to thickness.

By the time you finish working back in this routine, your biceps will be warmed up and slightly pumped up, so it's logical to work biceps next. Notice that there is no barbell curl in this routine because it is hard on the inner elbows. My years of training have proven to me that the best way to train biceps is with dumb bells. When you curl with DBs you can also supinate or turn your wrist outward on the way up, giving you an extra contraction you don't get with a barbell.

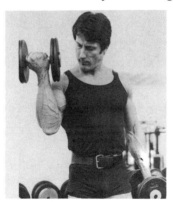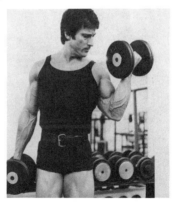

Alternate DB curl replaces barbell curl as it is a lot easier on the inner elbow. Curl completely up and down with one DB before curling the other DB, rotating your wrist outward (supinating) as you curl upward and turn your wrist slightly away from your body at the top of the movement.

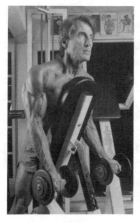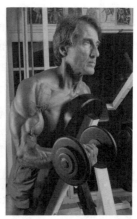

Face down incline DB curl is a great exercise because your biceps reach peak contraction at the very top of the movement. It is very important for biceps development not to relax the biceps at the top of the movement but to tense them instead. Then lower the DBs slowly to the starting position.

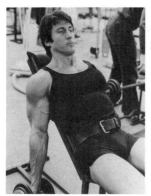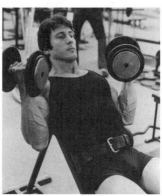

Incline DB curl allows the biceps to reach peak contraction about 2/3rds of the way up on the curl since you are in a reclining position. This exercise, however, gives a good stretch to the biceps when done correctly. Keep your upper arms anchored to your sides and tense the biceps as you turn your wrists slightly away from the body at the top of the movement.

It's very important to keep the wrists straight when curling. If you turn your wrist in towards your body as you curl, you contract your forearms at the expense of your biceps. This is why some people have been unable to develop their biceps. These same people almost always have well developed forearms. I spent the first ten years of my bodybuilding career curling this way until I learned this technique from Arnold Schwarzenegger when we trained together from 1969 to 1972.

Forearms are the final muscle group to work in this routine, and because you've actually been working them indirectly with your back and bicep training by gripping the weights, two exercises are usually sufficient to develop the forearms. I like to super-set barbell reverse curl with wrist curl (do both exercises without resting) because I get a better pump this way and my workout goes faster. These two exercises work opposite parts of the forearm.

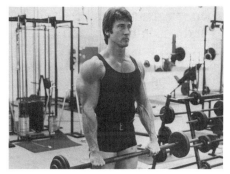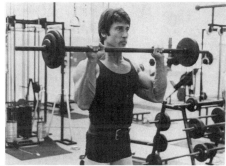

Reverse curl works the top part of the forearm. Grip the bar with your palms facing your body and curl the weight up to your chin and without pausing, lower the bar slowly until your arms are completely straight.

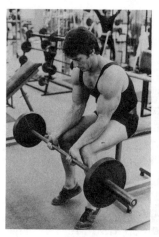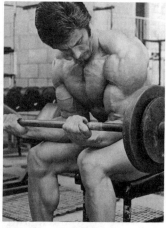

Wrist curl trains the underside of the forearm. Using a thumbless grip, let the bar roll down your hands into your fingers and then roll it rapidly back up to starting position. You'll get a better effect if you use a barbell with a thick diameter sleeve, as it is harder to grip. A few light sets of this exercise at the beginning of your workout is good for sore elbows. As your forearms get stronger, you lessen the chance of elbow and wrist injuries.

HOW TO PROGRESS: I keep my repetitions between 8 and 12 on back work, between 10 and 15 on biceps, and 12 to 20 on forearm training. When I first start this workout, I do 2 sets of each exercise for as long as I continue to feel some soreness the day following the session. Then I move to 3 sets of each exercise and stay at this level until one month before I want to reach a physical peak, at which time I move to 4 sets of each exercise. I use this system of adding sets on the leg as well as the chest, shoulder and tricep workouts.

I usually go heavier with each set and at the same time decrease the reps. I jump 5 to 10 pounds on barbell and machine exercises, and 2 & 1/2 to 5 pounds on dumb bell exercises. This increases strength and adds size to the muscles. If you're not interested in strength increases, you can use the same weight on each set, or even decrease the weight if you are resting little between sets. A good pace is to complete a set followed by a stretch every two minutes.

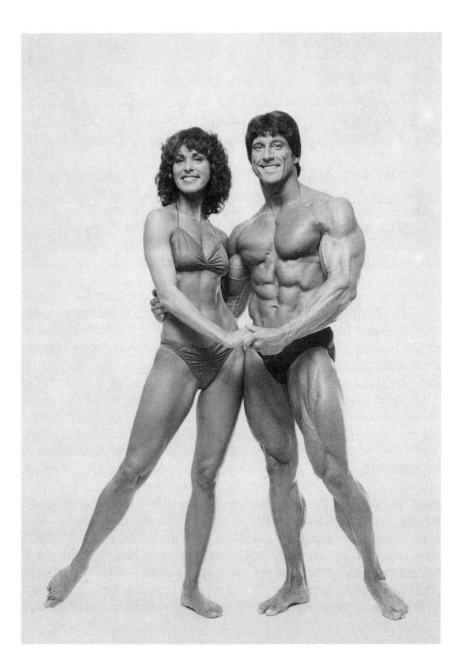

CHRISTINE AND FRANK, 1979

DAY 2: THIGHS, CALVES

Thighs
> LEG EXTENSION & one leg back stretch
> LEG CURL & one leg up stretch
> ERECT SQUAT & one leg back stretch
> LUNGE & one leg up stretch
> STAIRCLIMBER (2 to 5 minutes at a fast pace)

Calves
> STANDING CALF RAISE & calf stretch
> SEATED CALF RAISE & calf stretch
> DONKEY CALF RAISE & calf stretch

In this routine it is possible to begin your workout with either thighs or calves. The criteria I use for which choice I make is two fold. Since thigh work takes much more energy than calf work, if my pre-workout meal is still not fully digested by the time I begin training, I will start with calves. The other reason for starting with either thighs or calves is to specialize on either bodypart.

The priority principle states that what gets trained first gets trained hardest because you pay better attention to what you are doing at the beginning of your workout. So if you want bigger calves, then start with calf work--or if you want to gain weight, start with thigh work because the thighs are the biggest muscle group in the body. I found that when I added an extra inch to my thigh measurement, my bodyweight went up ten pounds. I always increase the weight by 10 pounds on each successive set of thigh exercises, keeping my repetitions in the 10 to 15 range with the negative slower than the positive.

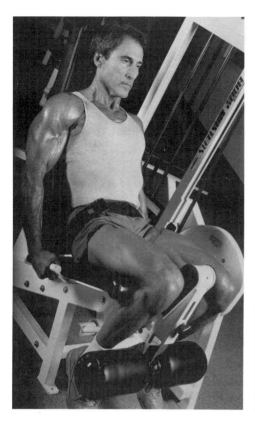

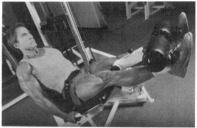

Leg extension is essential to do before squatting to warm up the knees and pump up the quadriceps or frontal thigh muscles. Leg extension is a must for defining the quads: vastus internus, medialus, and externus. Keep the reps between 10 and 15 and always lower the weight (negative phase) more slowly than you raised it (positive phase). You'll need a good leg extension machine for this one, and although the version I use, the Nautilus single chain, is no longer produced, I have found the latest **Body Masters** Leg Extension to be as good and it is capable of more adjustments. Combination leg extension-leg curl machines are usually not as good because the groove or pathway of each exercise is different. However, I have discovered a fantastic combo leg extension/curl unit with a great groove that is knee friendly by **Pro Industries**. The one leg back stretch is done after each set of leg extensions and is held for 15 seconds to stretch the quadriceps.

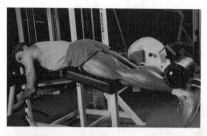

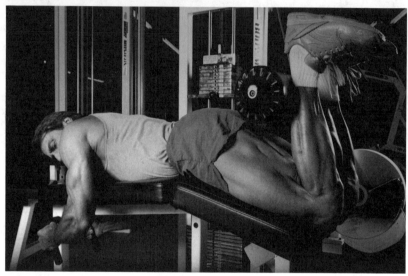

Leg curls are done at this point to pump up the leg biceps or hamstrings. This provides a cushioning or rebound effect when squatting erect, because the leg biceps help you recover out of the low position in the squat when the upper body is erect. I don't mean you should bounce out of the low position of the squat because this can be very dangerous. I prefer the bent back leg curl machine as the buttocks have a tendency to raise up as the leg curl is done. Leg curls also help warm up the backs of the knees and work the lower back and calves as well. The one leg up stretch is done following each set of leg curls, giving a terrific stretch to the hamstrings as well as the lower back.

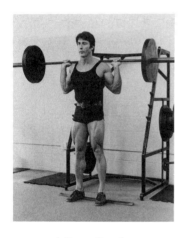
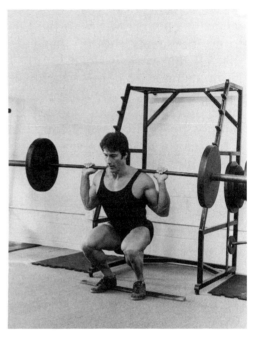

After the knees are warmed up, it's time for **squatting**. The best way to squat for maximum thigh development is with the upper body erect or perpendicular (at a 90 degree angle) to the floor. My squats with barbell on back were always fairly erect, except when the weight got heavier. This is why heavy squats gave me thick spinal erector muscle development. My lower back helped me recover out of the low position of the squat since my upper body was leaning forward. Squatting with upper body thrust forward also builds the waist as well as the buttocks. It is also very hard on the knees since they become compressed from being forced into a position well in front of the toes at the bottom of the movement. I feel that everyone who does heavy squats will eventually be forced to change the way they do this important exercise.

THE LEG BLASTER

I stopped regular barbell squatting in 1983 after incurring these problems from years of regular heavy squats. Since then, I have been squatting with the Leg Blaster, which enables me to do full squats with my hands free and upper body erect so that all the work is done by my thighs. I get a tremendous pump using a weight less than half of what I formerly used in the regular squat. The Leg Blaster has replaced barbell squat, front squat, hack squat, and leg presses in my thigh workouts. Simply by changing my foot positions, I can get the same effect as these movements without the pain, discomfort, and risk of injury.

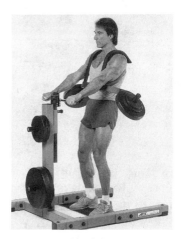

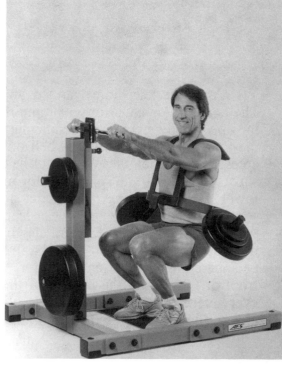

Women who want to reduce their hips and thighs should never squat with a barbell. Except for high repetition sissy squats with the upper body leaning backward with little or no weight, squats of any kind build the thighs even when done for high repetitions. Sissy squats are another exercise that can be done effectively with the Leg Blaster, with or without the shoulder harness.

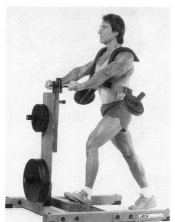
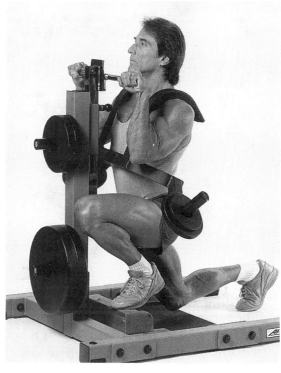

The Leg Blaster is a great way to do **lunges** as it provides good balance, making it unnecessary to use much weight. Lunges work the entire thigh and buttock area, but may be hard on the knees unless you take a step up to a block about 12 inches high. Be sure to lunge in deeply, almost sitting on your heel. Do all the reps for one leg before you go to the other leg.

Finish off the thigh routine with **stairclimber** as fast as you can go for 2 minutes, tensing the thighs at the top of each rep.

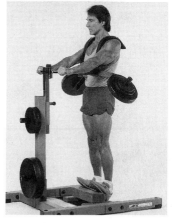
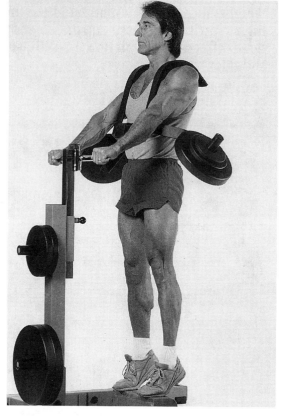

Standing calf raise is a good exercise to start calf work with, either using a standing calf machine or the Leg Blaster, which is excellent for calf raises. You'll need a calf block to stand on to allow your heels to stretch below the plane of the floor to full work the lower calf. Pause for a half second at the top of the calf raise to maximize contraction in the calves. I work up in weight on each set on all my calf exercises and do 3 sets of 15 to 25 reps. I prefer high reps on calf raises as it gives me a great burn necessary for growth. You must get a burn on every set of calf raises if you want your calves to grow! Do the calf stretch for 15 seconds after each set.

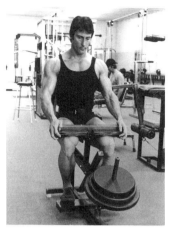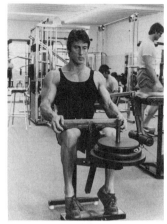

Seated calf raise which should be done after the Achilles tendon is fully warmed up. This exercise works the soleus, the large muscle underneath the gastrocnemius. Be sure to pause for one half second at the top of the seated calf raise for a maximum contraction. Don't use too much weight so you can stretch low in the movement and work the lower calf. Seated raises are especially good for the outer calf.

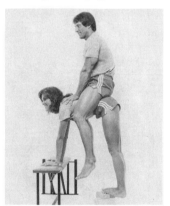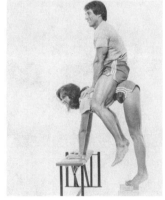

Donkey calf raise is my final exercise for calves. It is one of the very best calf movements, and can be done with a partner sitting on your lower back, or with a Nautilus multi purpose machine. I used this exercise exclusively for my calf training for the 1978 Mr. Olympia Contest with my partner holding a 50 pound plate for 8 non-stop sets of 20 to 25 reps.

DAY 3 - CHEST, SHOULDERS, TRICEPS

Chest
    30 DEGREE INCLINE DB PRESS & Doorway Stretch
    75 DEGREE INCLINE DB PRESS & Doorway Stretch
    or OVERHEAD PRESS MACHINE
    DB FLY & Doorway Stretch
    DB PULLOVER & 1 arm shoulder stretch

Triceps
    PRESSDOWN & arms back stretch
    CLOSE GRIP BENCH PRESS & arms back stretch
    I ARM DB EXTENSION & 1 arm shoulder stretch

Shoulders
    BENT OVER DB REAR DELT RAISE & rear delt str.
    DB SIDE RAISE & rear delt stretch

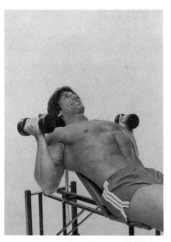 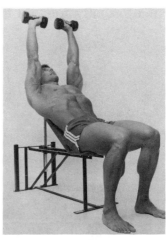

30 degree incline DB press works the upper pectorals and front deltoids. Be sure to turn the dumb bells so your palms face each at the bottom of the movement so you can get a deep stretch for the outer pecs. Exhale as you push the DBs to finish position stopping just short of lockout, keeping tension on the upper pecs.

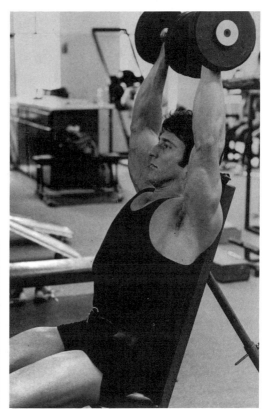

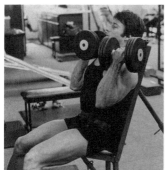

75 degree incline DB press works higher on the upper pecs around the clavicle area and provides a great deal of front deltoid work. It is more of a front deltoid exercise but this is a good place to do it--while the pressing muscles are still strong and before the triceps are too pumped up. Pressing on the overhead press machine can be substituted for this exercise. There are two types of pressing machines: those that move in a straight line and those that move in an arc away from the body. I find the straight line movement works deltoids more, while the arc movement works upper pecs as well as front delts. I prefer the arc press, my favorite movement being the **Soloflex** front press using additional weights loaded on the pressing bar, as this causes the least amount of stress on my shoulder joints and gives me a great pump as well.

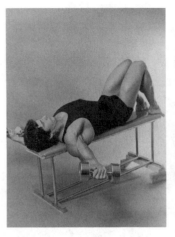 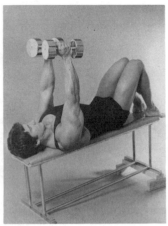

Dumb bell fly works the outer pecs and the deeper you lower the dumb bells, the more outer pec you work. Be sure to do the doorway stretch after each set of these first three exercise, as it stretches the entire pec and front delt region.

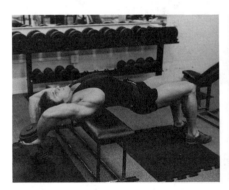 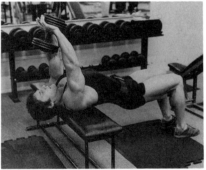

Dumb bell pullover gets the anterior serratus muscles, the ribcage, and the lower pecs. It will also really pump up the posterior triceps and that's why I like to do tricep work right afterwards. One arm shoulder stretch done between sets will help you get a deep stretch in the pullover. The **Nautilus** Plate Loaded Pullover Machine is a good substitute for this exercise.

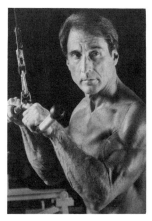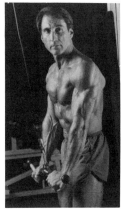

Pressdown works all three heads of the triceps and warms up the elbows. Be sure to hold the lockout for a half second on each rep, tensing the triceps hard before you return slowly to starting position.

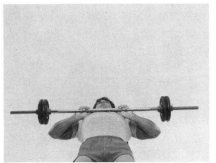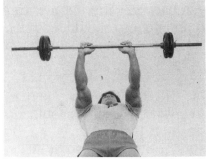

Close grip bench press with hands 12 inches apart and elbows pointing outward work the outer triceps as well as the inner pecs. This exercise can be done with an Olympic bar, cambered or EZ curl bar, or a Smith Machine. Be sure to lower the weight very slowly to the chest and press up until the elbows are almost locked out.

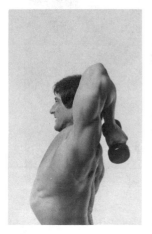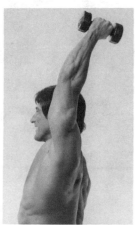

One arm dumb bell extension is my favorite for the posterior tricep providing you get a deep stretch at the bottom of the movement. On both close grip bench press and 1 arm dumb bell extension, don't lock out at the top of the movement--you'll get a better pump this way. Hold on to a support so you can lean back slightly in order to get a very deep stretch. Be sure to do one arm shoulder stretch between sets to loosen up your shoulder so you can stretch low with the dumb bell.

So far this routine has worked the pressing muscles involved in chest, shoulder and triceps movements. Now finish off the routine with DB raises to complete your shoulder work. Since the front delts have already been thoroughly worked with the incline presses, all that needs to be done are rear and side deltoids.

You may have noticed that this routine can be performed with dumb bells on all but two exercises (pressdown and close grip bench press), making it very easy to do in a home gym. It's always nice to have a complete set of dumb bells to get the best workout in the shortest time. My new dumb bells from **Advanced Free Weight Systems** have 2 and 1/2 pound increments from 5 to 45 pounds and 5 pound increments from 50 to 65 pounds.

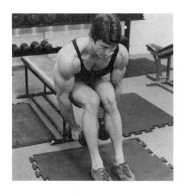 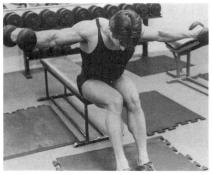

Bent over dumb bell rear delt raise is the standard for the rear delts. It's important not to use too heavy a weight or else you might work the trapezius more than the rear deltoids. Also, turn the back ends of the dumb bells slightly upward at the top of the movement, keeping the dumb bells parallel to the floor. Follow up with the rear delt stretch between sets.

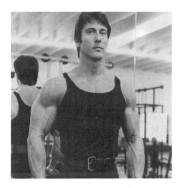 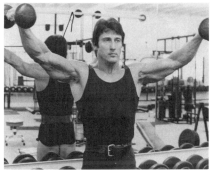

Dumb bell side raise is a great movement for the lateral delts. This exercise can also be done with one dumb bell at a time, since one dumb bell provides good deltoid isolation and is easier on the neck and trapezius. Two dumb bells make the exercise quicker and more expedient if you have no shoulder injuries. Be sure to bring the dumb bell directly to your side not to the front when returning to starting position or else you'll work more traps than deltoids.

How to Progress - This workout gives a great pump and should be done without much rest between sets--knock off a set and a stretch every two minutes. I like to keep my reps between 8 and 12, doing three sets and increasing the weights 2 & 1/2 to 5 pounds on the dumb bell exercises and 5 to 10 pounds on the barbell and machine exercises. As in all exercises my negative is slower than my positive movement, especially on the pressing exercises.

ABDOMINAL WORK

I usually work abs at the end of my workouts, but sometimes when I really want to specialize on them I will work them at the start of the session. This way I pay more attention to them. Make sure your pre-workout meal is well digested if you decide to train abs this way. The simplest ab workout includes an exercise for lower abdominals, one for upper abs, and one for sides or obliques. I also like to do a few sets of **hyperextension** to keep my lower back strong.

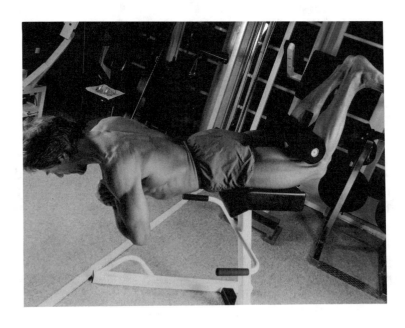

Leg Raise - 3 or 4 sets of 20 to 25 reps
Crunches - 3 or 4 sets of 20 to 25 reps
Seated Twist - 100 reps to each side non-stop
Hyperextension - 2 sets of 15 to 20 reps

Here is a more advanced abdominal program which you can use after being on the above program for at least one month: Do 3 or 4 super-sets (2 exercises in a row without stopping) of 25 to 50 reps each exercise. This saves time and increases your pulse rate, giving you an aerobic effect.

Leg raise supersetted with crunches
Knee-ups supersetted with partial incline sit-up
Seated twist supersetted with hyperextension.

AEROBICS

Do at least 12 minutes or up to 30 minutes of aerobic exercise at the end of your workout. On leg day this can be stationary bike or treadmill, or you can continue stairclimber for a longer period of time. On Back day do rowing and on Chest day airdyne or rowing.

EXERCISE MACHINES VS. FREE WEIGHTS

I'm often asked which is better, free weights or exercise machines? One form of exercise is not better than the other, as they are both excellent forms of training, but they are different: With free weights, that is barbells and dumb bells, a great deal of muscular coordination is required to keep the weights moving in the pathway of optimum resistance. This pathway is called the groove and keeping the weight in the groove is the most effective way to get a good pump. Free weight exercises, especially those with dumb bells, are a balancing act and take time to learn to do the movement in perfect form. All parts of your body can be worked effectively with free weights. Given barbells, dumb bells, adjustable flat to incline bench, overhead and low pulleys, squat racks or Leg Blaster, leg extension, and leg curl, you can do just about everything.

Weight machines didn't begin to gain popularity until the early 1970's when the first Nautilus machines were introduced. Today there are many equipment companies producing incredible exercise machines, and there are new inventions and improvements all the time. Machines are fun, require less skill to use because the groove is built in, and tend to isolate specific muscle groups. They are great for people just learning to do weight training and people who have injuries which restrict them from doing certain free weight movements. Here are the machine equivalents of free weight exercises:

FREE WEIGHT	MACHINE EQUIVALENT
Wide grip chin-ups	Lat machine pulldowns
Barbell row, T bar row	Low cable row or Seated row machine
1 arm dumb bell row	1 arm cable row
Preacher bench curl	Curling machine
Bench press	Vertical bench press machine
Incline press	Incline press or Smith machine
Overhead press	Universal or Soloflex press
Dumb bell fly	Pec deck
Dumb bell pullover	Nautilus plate loaded Pullover machine
Parallel dips	Dip machine
DB side raise	Lateral raise machine
Bent over DB rear delt raise	Nautilus torso row
Barbell squat	Leg Blaster, Smith machine, or Leg press
Donkey calf raise	Nautilus multi purpose machine
Standing calf machine	Leg Blaster calf raise
Sit-ups	Abdominal machine*
Seated twist	Rotary torso machine*

* can cause lower back injury if heavy weights are used.

In general, free weights provide a more global effect, that is, you feel the effect of the exercise in a larger area of your body. Machines are expensive compared to free weights, usually ranging from $1000 to $5000 per machine. Every free weight exercise has its machine equivalent, so if you can't do an essential free weight movement due to injury, you may be able to use a machine and obtain similar benefits.

THE RIGHT EQUIPMENT

When it comes to choosing free weight exercises versus machines, my rule is "if it hurts, don't do it". I'm not talking about the over used and abused bodybuilding metaphor "no pain, no gain", I'm speaking of joint pain, which should be avoided at all costs. Over the years, I've had to eliminate some free weight exercises from my program for this very reason. With machines, you are less likely to wobble out of the groove and get injured. If it weren't for machines I would have a lot of undeveloped bodyparts. Let me give you some examples:

Barbell bench press is a very popular exercise especially for beginners. But as you continue to do heavier and heavier bench presses, especially with a wide grip in loose form, you may incur shoulder and pec injuries. Instead of bench press there are now bench press machines available which work the pecs and take some of the stress off the shoulders. Parallel dips are a great movement which require only a pair of parallel bars and maybe some weights to attach around your waist if you are strong. After years of doing dips, I now use a dip machine because regular dips just hurt too much. Dumb bell flys are unexcelled for developing the outer pecs, but due to shoulder injury, I now use a pec deck and get great results. Because of shoulder injuries, I do less overhead pressing with dumb bells --instead, I rely on the arc movement of the **Soloflex** for front press. Because they stress the inner elbow, barbell curls are out, various kinds of dumb bell curls are in. I especially like my recently acquired **Panatta Curling Machine**, which is best machine for curls on the market.

To minimize stress on the lower back it is important to wear a lifting belt on all standing movements like curls, squats, rowing, and all overhead lifting as well as deadlifting. The best most comfortable belt I have found is the **Valeo Belt**. Its cloth/velcro design fits snug around the waist and its not too thick design provides belt contact points in key areas -- unlike most thick leather belts which are too stiff, too wide in the back, and the buckle digs into your waist. Not so with Valeo.

Leg work in general requires more machines than upper body training because the legs have fewer articulations than arm movements do. A leg extension and leg curl machine are absolutely essential for maximum thigh development. exercises. For a home gym I like the **Pro Industries combination Leg Extension/ Leg Curl** the best. It provides a superior movement in both exercises and takes up less space than its more expensive individual counterparts. This combination unit costs under $2000 as compared to over $2000 for <u>either</u> an individual leg extension or leg curl machine.

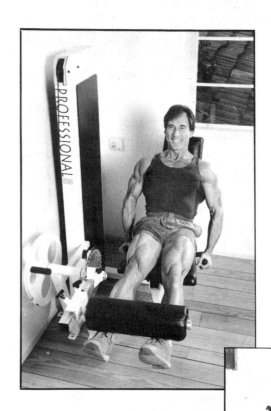

Instead of barbell squats, I use the **Leg Blaster** for squatting with the upper body perfectly erect to isolate the thighs. I also use it for standing calf raises to eliminate pressure on the shoulders which standing calf machines create.

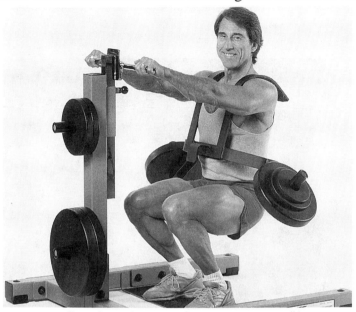

I use a **Soloflex** for my front presses. Slow negatives with added barbell plates give me a tremendous pump.

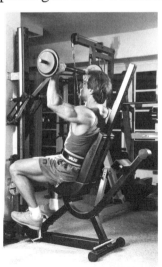

People with chronically sore lower backs would do well to use the "**Back Revolution**" on a regular basis for hanging upside down for lower back traction as well as hyperextensions. This device is the second generation "Orthopod" and is much better made. It is safer and more effective than "gravity boots".

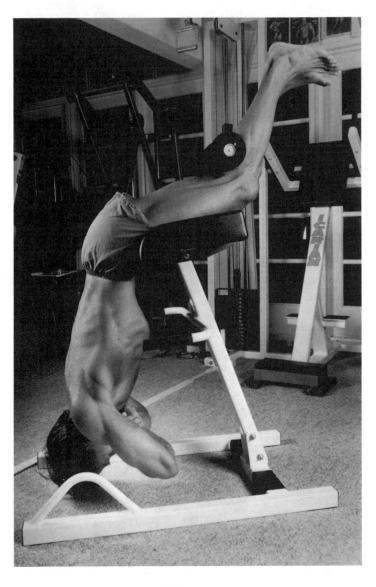

Preference HRT 2000 Semi-Recumbent Bike is my choice for a stationary aerobic bicycle. It is real easy on the groin and buttocks, and provides superior resistance not only for the frontal thigh, but also for the hamstrings which regular stationary bikes miss. The semi-recumbent position is like a horizontal leg press and the tension can be adjusted manually to make it feel like a heavy alternate leg press. It requires no electrical plug in and has a good selection of programs plus a built in heart rate monitor. Everybody who has trained in my Zane Experience Gym loves this bike.

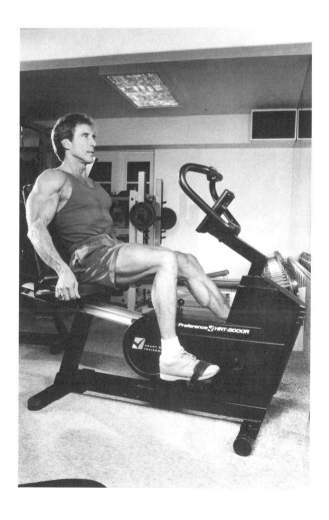

For home gym training, I use the **Precor M 9.4 E/L Personal Treadmill** for my indoor walk/run workouts. I love program 9 which can be set to change from 2 degrees decline to 12 degrees incline automatically every minute. Decline treadmill works the frontal thighs and tibialis and incline treadmill works the buttocks, hamstrings, and really works the calves like nothing else! **Precor's C 964 Treadmill** is the very best treadmill for home as well as heavy health club use. It feels like you are running on a cushioned rubberized track because the platform gives as your feet hit it.

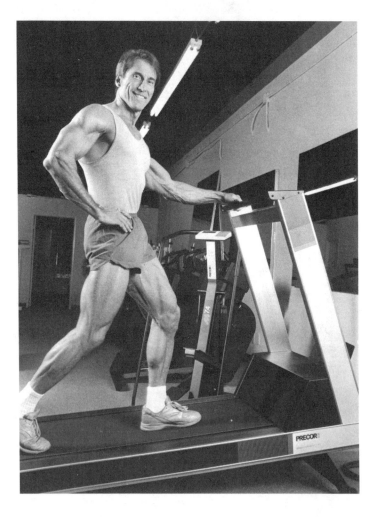

The new **Concept II Rowing Ergometer Model C** is the best aerobic rowing machine by far and costs only $700. I row 500 to 2500 meters at the end of my upper body workouts for more definition in my back, waist, shoulders, and arms.

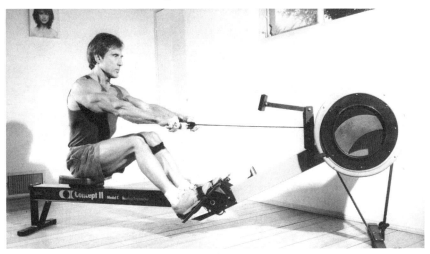

In general, I've noticed a trend away from using barbell exercises as I've grown older. About the only barbell exercises I still do are wrist curl and reverse wrist curl. Everything else is a cable, dumb bell or machine equivalent. The problem with barbells is that when you grip a barbell, you lock your arms into a fixed position that can be hard on the elbows, shoulders, and wrists, especially when a wide grip is used. Other exercises which involve pulling (wide grip chin ups, barbell rows, and pulldowns with a straight bar) as well as pushing (barbell bench press, press behind neck, and overhead press) can injure the elbows, shoulders and wrists because the hands cannot rotate freely. It's much easier to do all pushing and pulling movements with dumb bells or a curved bar with a grip where the palms face each other. I've changed to this kind of grip on all my pulldowns and rowing motions.

In order to keep working out the rest of your life, it's important to avoid injuries as you progress in your training. Chapter 7 explores the psychosomatic aspects of injury.

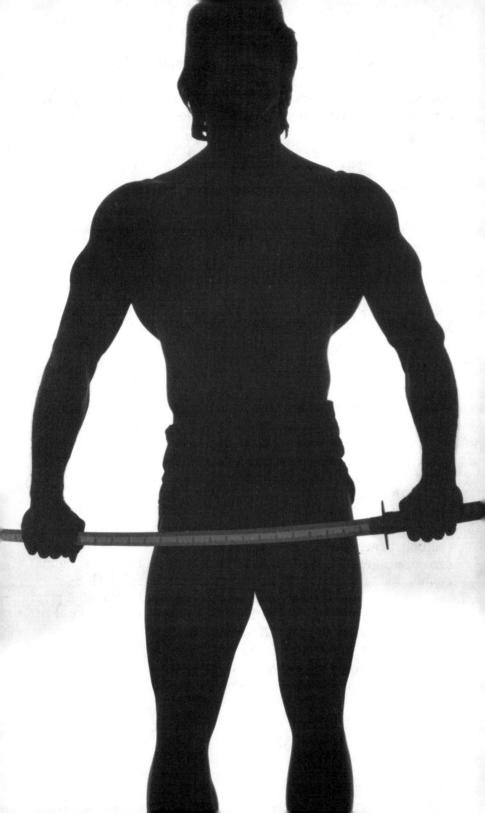

CHAPTER 7
PREVENTING AND HEALING INJURIES

Once there was a schoolmaster who loved to spend his holidays by himself in the mountains. One day he heard church bells, but since there was no church nearby, he looked around and was astonished when he saw a group of people in Sunday clothes moving along on a path in front of his hut which had not been there before. He followed them and came to a little wooden church which was also new to him. He was very impressed by the old pastor's sermon, but it seemed unconventional.

After the service, the schoolmaster was invited to the pastor's house, where the daughter asked him if he would be the old pastor's successor when he died. The daughter said that she would give the schoolmaster a year to decide. Afterwards, he felt puzzled, and then the matter slipped his mind.

The following year he was again in his mountain hut and noticing that the roof was weathering away, he climbed up with his axe to do some repair work. Suddenly he saw the pastor's daughter coming down the path in front of his hut. Seeing him, she asked if he was willing to accept the pastorship. He replied, "I cannot answer for it to God and my conscience, so I must refuse." At that moment the girl disappeared and he inadvertently brought the axe down upon his knee, with the result that he was crippled for the rest of his days.

Scandinavian folk tale (1)

It was two weeks before the 1974 Mr. Olympia competition and I was training furiously to get as "cut up" -- that is, to develop as much muscular definition--as possible. Returning home after my workout, I noticed that three bottles of drinking water were outside the door. As I picked one up, the bottom fell out, cutting my index finger severely. I rushed to the hospital, got it stitched up, and spent my final two weeks of training for the competition with my finger in a splint.

I've experienced my share of injuries, accidents, and illness during my training career, so I feel I know a little about their nature. One element these mishaps all have in common is that they happened to me. Since I was the one who experienced them, I must have something to do with their occurrence--not God, not the devil, but ME! The first step, therefore, in healing is to ask the question, "What part did I play in bringing this about?" My own healing process didn't begin until I took responsibility for creating the problem.

If you practice self observation, you will eventually discover that intention precedes movement. Before you move a muscle there is the volition to do it. There is a choice, but this choice is usually not made consciously--it is made automatically and unconsciously. Either you choose consciously and intentionally or your conditioning and belief system chooses for you. And indeed, this is the case with accident, injury, and illness. Your lack of awareness chooses and you suffer unnecessarily.

Another incident occurred after I had spent two weeks on bodybuilding tour in Japan. I had not trained the way I wanted, so immediately upon arriving home, I went to the gym. My head was reeling from jet-lag but I went over to the bench press anyway and pulled off a 35 pound plate for my first set. I didn't notice the sharp edged 10 pound plate in front of it and it slid off and cut my toe through my shoe. I rushed to the hospital and before long I was in stitches again. Since I had refused to listen to my body's message to rest as manifested by the jet-lag, I paid the price.

Both of my accidents accomplished the bodybuilding goal to "get cut up" in a literal sense. Associated with every injury or illness is such a metaphor, and part of the healing process results in being made aware of these negative metaphorical implications. Of course, most people heal anyway even though unaware of these metaphorical connections, but it takes longer and they remain ignorant of the relation between injury and metaphor.

Your body always gets its way. Through experience we learn the difference between making excuses not to train (rationalization) and listening to our body (wisdom or experience) which tells us our body needs a rest. Over-training can suppress the body's immunity to infection (2). If you are feeling tired and over-trained, don't say "I feel like I'm coming down with something". Instead say "I feel like my body is fighting fatigue and needs to rest". You'll suffer less if you choose and use the right words to express yourself.

THE POWER OF POSITIVE SPEAKING

About 2500 years ago, Plato called the thinking process "internal dialog" or the ongoing conversation we carry on with ourself. Modern psychologists call this internalized form of speech "self talk" and agree it characterizes much of our thoughts. Concurrent with Plato's thinking about his internal dialog was the Buddha's expression "Our lives are shaped by our minds. We become what we think" (3). Since we think with words of inner dialog, and consequently become what we think, it makes sense to choose the best possible words to express ourselves.

Right speech is about the role words play in the creation of positive life experience. Since we use words to talk and think with, words become the structure of our thoughts as well as our speech. The words we repeat in thinking and talking become the tools of our creative expression: when thinking we express ourself to ourself, when talking we express ourself to others. Thought leads to speech. We "think up" what to say before we say it. Speech leads to action or behavior. We "talk up" what we do before we do it. Repetitive thoughts and speech mold our belief system and thus influence our behavior.

We also use figures of speech called metaphors as part of the thinking and speaking process. According to Aristotle, "Metaphor consists in giving the thing a name that belongs to something else" (4). Metaphor means expressing the unknown in terms of the familiar. It is impossible to think without metaphor and difficult to speak intelligently without using metaphors. But if we want the best results from our training, it's a good idea to retire outworn figures of speech from our thoughts and expression. This will help us avoid injury, accidents, and illness.

Of course the question arises, does the injury cause the metaphor, or does the metaphor cause the injury? It can work both ways. The relation between injury and metaphor is the same as the question, "Which came first, the chicken or the egg"? Both events are correlated: where you find one you find the other. We lost track of which came first long ago. Frederick Nietzsche writes:

> "The involuntariness of image and metaphor is the strangest of all: one no longer has any idea of what is an image and what is a metaphor; everything offers itself as the nearest, most obvious, simplest expression. It actually seems as if the things themselves approached and offered themselves as metaphors." (5)

Myths are metaphors, the word being derived from the Greek "mythos" meaning speech. Myths, however do not mean false beliefs, rationalizations, or excuses. Myth is an ennobling, symbolic, and meaningful interpretation of reality. Myths, folk tales, fairy tales and fables have been used throughout the history of civilization as a vehicle for conveying high level information. Don't confuse myth with personal fiction or an inaccurate belief system.

We all have false beliefs about exercise and the aging process and these seem to proliferate as we get older. Personal fiction such as "I'm too old to start exercising", "I keep junk food in the house for the kids", "I don't have time, money, energy, or the genetics for exercise", are all belabored excuses used by mature people as a rationalization for not training. The problem is, because they are repeated so often as part of the thinking and talking process, they have become indelibly etched in one's belief system. In effect they become true for the individual.

I am often asked the question, "How old will I be before I stop making bodybuilding progress?" I must admit that I don't know the answer to this question but I am curious to find out. If I were to tell people some age, this might become self-fulfilling prophecy. I would be creating my own false belief system. Instead, I keep training and practicing the bodybuilding way of life and observe what happens. Curiosity motivation is very powerful.

NEGATIVE BODY METAPHORS

Using metaphors which indicate false beliefs about the body and the aging process are dangerous because they can provoke unconscious suffering. The body suffers unnecessarily when we use it as a medium to express our anger, distaste, laziness. My experience has shown me that there is a correlation between injury, lack of progress, illness, and accidents with the metaphors we use to express ourselves. Such "negative body metaphors" litter the speech of the aging and seem to be reflected in the condition of their bodies.

Negative body metaphors have at least one of three characteristics:

1. They contain the word "Pain".
2. They are phrased as "that makes me _____".
3. They mention a part of the body or a function of the body such as, "I can't stand that".

By practicing self observation, you may discover that your mind often takes what you say literally and allows your body to act on it. As a result, you may unconsciously behave in such a way as to make your figures of speech come true.

I've observed in myself as well as in others that the figures of speech people use are accurate descriptions of what's ailing them. I know of people with injured backs telling others to "get off my back", nauseated people telling of experiences that "make them sick", and clumsy people who "can't handle situations". Not only are their lives unpleasant, but they are creating unnecessary suffering in their bodies. Be kind to your body by finding a better way of speaking!

Wrong speech involves the use of "pun" or play on words. "You're a pain in the neck" refers to a person or situation you don't like. But a pain in the neck is also something physical and very real. I was guilty of using this negative body metaphor in my past and by unconsciously using my body to express my dislike, I found my neck hurting most of the time. Such pains don't just magically or mystically occur. We create them with our actions. I remember once going to the gym and doing heavy power cleans without warming up after having complained about people who were "a pain in the neck". This taught me to listen to what I said and how I said it and then observe my subsequent physical actions and reactions. I learned that my past history was stored in my body, and since history tends to repeat itself, it was up to me to create my future according to my real bodybuilding goals.

As we grow older what usually happens in the normal course of human development is body entropy, which I feel is connected with the unnecessary use of negative body metaphors and negative beliefs about aging and exercise. Negative body metaphors show negative self-conception. This results in, or is at least correlated to, the body developing ailments which hinder bodybuilding progress. Since we also get smarter with age-- "If I only knew then what I know now"-- we should realize how we impose barriers by self-limiting thoughts, words, and behaviors. Intention always precedes action. Only until we become aware of how we predetermine our actions by what we think and what we say, can we take steps to change these erroneous attitudes.

COMMONLY USED NEGATIVE BODY METAPHORS

Here is a list of negative body metaphors people often use in describing their experiences and the consequences they may lead to (6):

"Oh my aching back"	back pain
"No one ever backs me up"	back problems
"Get off my back"	poor posture
"Pain in the ass"	buttocks problems
"I can't handle that"	hand and grip problems
"I can't grasp that"	can't hold on
"Foul taste in my mouth"	bad breath, poor taste
"Nothing moves me"	laziness, constipation
"I can't stand that"	poor thigh/calf development
"I don't want to hear it"	hearing and ear problems
"I don't want to see that"	vision and eye problems
"I can't face that"	ugliness, facial problems
"Shouldering a heavy load"	posture/shoulder issues
"I can't stomach that"	indigestion, nausea
"Can't get it off my chest"	chest/breathing weakness
"I'm fed up"	poor appetite, overeating
"That's hard to swallow"	throat problems
"That makes my skin crawl"	rashes, pimples
"That's a headache"	headache, migranes
"Glutton for punishment"	over-training, overeating
"Something's eating me"	cancer
"That kills me","I wish I were dead"	death
"That pisses me off"	urinary problems

I almost killed myself with this last negative body metaphor. I used this expression frequently when I was feeling angry or resentful. Feeling angry one morning, I went to lie by my pool to get a tan, when the lawn chair slid into the pool and I severed my urethra internally, causing massive bleeding. A catheter was inserted and I learned another meaning for being pissed off. This incident cost me my fourth straight Mr. Olympia victory and taught me the connection between negative body metaphors and real life suffering.

I began to learn how to use right speech to overcome angry feelings. Up to this point, I had been increasing my feelings of anger by continuing to say angry things. This obsessive clinging to my experience of anger left me tired and debilitated. By speaking more kindly, I began to think more kindly, which ultimately led to feeling more relaxed. I also learned to be less judgmental of others by using the word "unskillful" in place of "bad" or "stupid" (7).

Wrong speech is often expressed as self-invalidation. Negative expressions such as "I never do anything right", "I can't do it", I'll always be fat", "I'm stupid", all perpetuate a lack of confidence and set you up for failure. Not only do others hear your self-degredation, but you hear it as well and store it in your memory. These invalidations become part of your belief system. So if you hear yourself saying such negative expressions, stop and say "erase that". Then rephrase your sentiments with something positive. Your body believes every word you say.

Whenever others attempt to invalidate you, erase their negative comments in the same manner. Simple word exchanges are effective: rather than saying "He bugs me" substitute "I'm having a challenging time with him". You'll find it's much easier to be a success when you associate with positive people. It's important to seek out such acquaintances. But since the right company isn't always possible, it's important to be mindful of practicing right speech at all times.

Powerless speech includes expressions which in effect tell the world that you have no control, no power, no responsibility; the devil made you do it! Powerless speech is an admission that life just happens to you-- that you have no choice in determining the outcomes of events in your life. There is something out there in the environment that always "makes you" behave in the only way that is possible for you. This is the attitude of a victim of circumstance not a creator of positive life experiences.

While it is true that there are events in life we have little to do with, such as we have no say in who are parents are, we do have more choice in life than many people realize. This is not an easy fact to realize for people who constantly set up aversive behavioral outcomes by what they say.

TRANSFORMING POWERLESS SPEECH

Here are some examples of how to transform powerless speech by substituting positive expressions: (8)

INSTEAD OF SAYING:	SAY INSTEAD:
That makes me angry	I feel angry, I make me angry
I have to	I choose to
I need	I want
I can't	I don't, I won't
I doubt	I wonder
I'm too tired to exercise	I'm tired and I choose to rest
I am nervous	I am excited
It's boring	I prefer to
I'll try to	I'll do it
I always	I sometimes
"I always make errors"	"I sometimes make errors"
I sometimes	I always
"I sometimes can relax"	"I always can relax"
I never	It would be better when
I should	I could
I ought to	I would
I hope	I expect, I trust
I think	I know that
I'm sorry	I'm concerned
I'm worried that	I wonder if
It's difficult	It's challenging
It's frustrating	It's complicated but challenging
I'll rest if I finish	I'll rest when I finish

Right speech is both saying what you mean as well as meaning what you say. It is a powerful influence on behavior. The energy we conserve by not investing in negative thoughts and wrong speech is expressed in positive actions which help us reach our goals. When you transform your speech you will transform your body.

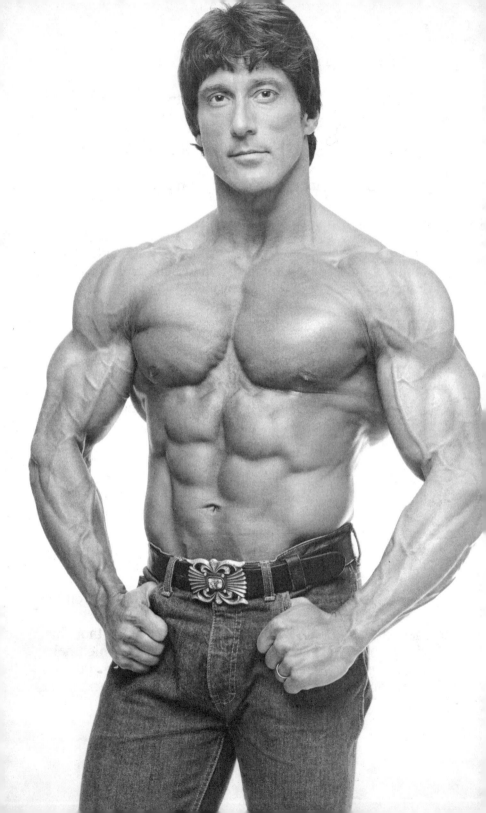

THE POWER PHRASE

Negative speech and self-talk are transformed into affirmative speech which lead to positive behaviors by the POSITIVE AFFIRMATION or POWER PHRASE. Here are some examples:

I am strong and creative
I am relaxed and centered
I am energetic and full of vitality
I grow stronger and more powerful every day
Everything works when I let it
I am inventing my body right now
I am certain I will succeed
What I say is true for me
I expect maximum progress
I am excited about my workout
I have stamina and endurance
I feel my waistline shrinking
I am experiencing my body's perfection
I will always get a good pump
A pump is a swell feeling
I will relax completely whenever I choose
When I train hard, people notice
I accept compliments graciously
I respond with ease and humor
Nutritious food always tastes good
I have plenty of energy for aerobic exercise
I am flexible and can stretch my limits
My path is my goal
I have already won
Next time I'm dreaming, I want to remember to
    recognize that I'm dreaming.
Am I dreaming or not?

These last two are lucid dream affirmations which are most effective when repeated before sleep, or when you wake up from sleep. As you persist in saying these affirmations with passive volition, you will also begin to say them when you are asleep and thereby initiate a lucid dream (see Chapter 12 on Dream-work).

Simply repeat your affirmation over and over again whenever you remember to do so during the day. The best times are when you are doing work that doesn't require your full attention, like driving a car, or in any situation in which you'd like to tune out incoming sounds. It's a good idea to start this practice immediately upon awakening in the morning as a meditation practice as described in Chapter 10. You will find that what you say is what you get!

It has been said that if a person speaks the truth long enough eventually his or her word becomes law. It's also true that your word will become law for you and result in negative outcomes even if you don't speak the truth. You've created yourself, your body, your mind, and your attitude exactly as you are today by how you thought, spoke, and behaved. As your words get repeated throughout your life, hopefully you will get to observe how these same words become law for you. And at the same time, with the consistent application of the techniques of right speech as I've outlined, you'll learn how the words of powerful people such as yourself become law for everyone else.

HEALING INJURIES

The steps to healing an injury are:

1. Take responsibility by not blaming someone or something else. What part did you play in the injury? You did it, you are experiencing it, no one else. How did you create this situation for yourself?

2. By paying attention to what you say and the words you use, find the negative body metaphor associated with the injury.

3. Begin to restructure your speech by substituting positive affirmations or power phrases for negative body metaphors.

4. Have a healing dream, where you become lucid, (that is, wake up in your dream and realize you are dreaming even though you are still asleep), take control, behave exceptionally, and heal.

Injuries are what stops you in making training progress. My best advice is to avoid injury in the first place. If you do get an injury, ask yourself "What can I still train?" Do what doesn't hurt and train around the injury. This is the best time to specialize on weakpoints. An injured shoulder shouldn't prevent you from doing extra abdominal and leg work.

An injury is a strong request or command by your body to get you to pay more attention to a particular bodypart. Injured wrists and elbows usually mean you need stronger forearms, and if this is the case, you should begin upper body workouts with light forearm exercises which don't hurt (my favorites are wrist curl and reverse wrist curl super-setted using a fat sleeved barbell). If your shoulders grind and click when you do presses or lateral raises, find movements where this doesn't happen (try warming up more and changing your grip so that your palms face each other while pressing). Spend more time stretching and warming up with lighter weights on the first set, and above all, KEEP THE INJURED AREA WARM WHILE TRAINING. If you have sore shoulders you shouldn't be training in a tank top in a cold gym.

I use two different linaments to keep joints warm during workouts, depending on the gym temperature. In cold weather, I rub "Eucalyptamint" (who now make a rub that smells like baby powder) into the area and then cover with a loose elastic bandage if it's your elbows, wrists, knees, or ankles, or a sweatshirt if it' your shoulders. In hot weather I apply "Heet" linament to the affected area (this preparation will heat up only if you are sweating so that your pores open up). Following your workout apply ice to the sore area and keep elevated.

After a game, a baseball pitcher immediately applies ice to his shoulder. Ice is also good before bed as it numbs the area thereby reducing pain and swelling and sets up a nice blood circulation for hours after the ice is removed. Getting a fresh blood supply into an injured area helps remove toxins and promotes healing. The best icepacks are **Polar Powder**--they provide a gradual longer lasting cold. These are simple precautions that can easily be followed by everyone who hurts.

For those injuries that don't seem to go away you might seek help from a chiropractor or physical therapist. I've found treatments like ultra-sound and low voltage pulsed micro-amp electrical stimulation to be helpful in healing stubborn injuries. Micro-current electrical neuromuscular stimulation or MENS, more closely approximates the natural bio-electrical currents in the body and therefore seems to enhance tissue repair, healing, and provide prolonged pain relief. (9) I also use higher voltage electric stimulation on the "tetanize" mode of my Amrex Muscle Stimulator (this is a continuous delivery of low threshold current, just enough to make the muscle twitch).

Other remedies like DMSO and buffered aspirin can also be helpful when used in moderation. However, I strongly recommend professional help for intense acute or prolonged chronic pain. Anti-inflammatory agents that must be prescribed by a medical doctor may be helpful if heat, ice, ultra-sound, or MENS do not provide sought after relief. But if damage is severe, surgical repair may be necessary.

If you are unlucky enough to need surgery, it's best to receive it form a surgeon who only does this type of operation. In 1983 I had rotator cuff surgery on my shoulder because of a bicycling accident, but I had to spend a year in rehabilitation building my shoulder back to normal.

THE HEALING DREAM

The night after this traumatic surgery I remember the dream that helped me change my attitude toward my healing:

Unfriendly people were chasing me and as I ran from them, I noticed that I only had one arm. After being pursued for some time and not wanting to run away any longer, I realized I was dreaming and decided that since this was my dream, I could do whatever I wanted. At that moment, my arm grew back and I discovered that I could fly. As I became airborn and rose above my pursuing adversaries, I felt a sense of freedom and pleasure in being able to soar among the clouds. After flying some distance and performing many fantastic aerial feats, I came upon a breathtaking view--a huge snowcapped mountain on the shore of the Pacific Ocean. As I hovered facing the mountain, I knew it was too steep to fly directly up the front and reach the top, so I flew around to the side of the lofty peak and discovered steps gradually winding up the mountain. I flew a few feet above the steps, ascending slowly to the very top of the mountain where I awoke in a beautiful garden paradise.

This dream marked the beginning of my recovery from the traumatic surgery and contained many valuable symbolic messages. Dreams can be kinesthetic experiences that help maintain body image and serve an emergency repair function, strengthening the body image when it is in flux. My body image as well as the healing process was threatened, as symbolized by my self perception of having only one arm and being pursued by unfriendly people. Growing a new arm was my dream's emergency repair function.

This was a flying dream that symbolized confidence and the feeling of success. The message for me was to have faith in the natural and gradual healing process and not to doubt my ability to "rise above" adverse life situations. I wasn't to attempt to "reach my peak" immediately--the slope was too steep and dangerous. Rather, by intentional exploration and discovery, I would find the route to the top--one with many gradual transitions which I would negotiate one step at a time. Eventually I would awaken at the top in "peak" condition.

Interpreting this dream helped me realize that it foretold what would later occur in my life. This was a pre-cognitive lucid dream (10) that gave me insight to change the way I trained: more exercise machines, lighter weights, slower repetitions. I did learn what it was like to start training as a real beginner. This helped me later on in my work as a trainer to understand and empathize with people who were beginning to get back into shape.

I also received some good advice from my surgeon: For rehabilitation, train the affected area every day with light weights, high reps, and STOP AT MILD DISCOMFORT. This good advice, along with gradual progressive weight-training and many years of muscle memory enable me to heal completely.

USE REST/PAUSE INSTEAD OF FORCED REPS

One way injuries can occur is when you push yourself beyond your limits and do forced reps. Forced reps means that someone else--a spotter--assists you to do a few more reps after you've reached failure in your set and can do no more repetitions on your own. This may be OK if done in correct form with a careful spotter, but many times people cheat and push or pull the weight up unevenly, causing injury.

A much better way to get the benefit of forced reps (which is deeper muscle stimulation, growth, and consequently, deeper soreness) is the "rest pause" system. Do as many reps as you can in perfect form, stop, rest 15 to 20 seconds, and then do 2 or 3 more reps, slowly in perfect form as before. You are in control at all times with rest pause and you will grow in personal power because you always accomplish what you set out to do. Instead of cheating or bouncing out reps in poor form, you do perfect reps only, and then complete your set with more perfect reps after a short rest.

I like to do slow negatives of 3 to 6 seconds in duration when I use the rest pause system. This is not a system you should use at all times--only when you are in the final few months of training to reach your absolute peak each year in your training season.

Obsession with heavy weights has much to do with injury. As I've grown older, I've been forced to use lighter weights in all my exercises. But at the same time, I've slowed down the speed of my repetitions so that my muscles interpret the weight as being heavier. There is way too much emphasis in the sport of bodybuilding on the amount of weight used in an exercise rather than on perfect form and movement. This obsession with big numbers is part of the bodybuilding inflation rampant throughout the years. It's much safer to pay attention to how an exercise feels in the muscles, not how heavy the weights are.

THE STAR METHOD

A great way to get feedback on your training as well to avoid injury is to keep a workout journal or diary in which you record each workout. To use the star method, write down each exercise, the weight you used and the number of reps you did with it for each set. When you do more weight for the same amount of reps or do more reps with the same weight on your last set of an exercise, put a star after the exercise. Work at scoring stars on about one-fourth to one-third of all your exercises in a workout. This is called the "weight star method" and will enable you to gradually build up your exercise poundages, gain strength and muscle, while at the same time minimize the risk of injury.

The other variation of the star method is the "time star method". Count how many total sets you do in a workout and how many minutes it takes you to complete your training. Next time, do the same amount of sets in less time, or more sets in the same amount of time. Time star will help you develop more muscular definition. Be sure not to decrease your weights to do this or you may lose muscle size.

In training for competition, I used the weight star method for about five months gradually building my poundages, and then the last month, I switched to the time star method for more definition. Another way you can use these two systems is to switch from the weight star to the time star whenever you find your workout going too slow from too long a rest period between sets, or if you are excessively sore or have injuries. The time star will jolt you out of your training doldrums, give you more definition, and make more efficient use of your workout time. When you want to again emphasize building size you can revert back to the weight star.

THE TRAINING DIARY

In order to use either star method, you must keep a training diary. Diaries help you keep track of your progress and give you feedback on the rate you are progressing in your training. I've found diaries to be invaluable motivational tools for enhancing bodybuilding progress because they make me more aware of how I'm progressing in my workouts. And because they emphasize awareness and control and reduce the risk of injury because of their gradual approach to progress, the star methods enhance training longevity.

To set up your training diary, list the exercises in your training program for the day. Then as you complete each set and stretch, write down the poundage you used and the reps you did with this poundage above it. Put a comma between each set, and a star at the end of each exercise when you score a weight star. Record the time you start and the time you finish your workout and the total amount of sets you did in your workout. Put a star at the end of your workout when you score a time star. See pages 282-283 for an example of the bodybuilding diary. Here is a sample page from my own training diary:

154

2-4-93 BACK, BICEPS, FOREARMS   START ABS, 10 AM

ABS PULLEY KNEE IN - 40 LBS - 4 sets 40 REPS

SUPER (INCLINE LEG RAISE ~ 3 × 50
SET   (CRUNCHES   ~ 3 × 50

       1 ARM CABLE CRUNCH - 80# 2 × 30 each side
       HYPEREXTENSION - 2 × 20

                                        REPS
                           12 10   9   WEIGHT
BACK (FRONT PULLDOWN - 160, 170, 180
SUPER   15 12   9   (2 arm
SET   (CROSSOVER BEHIND NECK - 50, 60, 70   lat stretch)

                        12 10   9
       LOW CABLE ROW - 150, 160, 170
                      10 10   9   (1 arm lat
       1 ARM DB ROW - 60, 65, 70   stretch)
                            12 11 10
       SEATED MACHINE ROW - 110, 120, 130

BICEPS
                             12 11   10
       DB CONCENTRATION CURL ~ 30, 32½, 35

       BISTAR CURL - 30 × 12 · 3 sets

SUPER (FACE DOWN INCLINE DB CURL - 27½ × 10 - 3 sets
SET   (PREACHER CABLE CURL ~ 70 × 10 - 3 sets
                                          (pronated arms
                                           back stretch)
FOREARMS

TRI   (REVERSE WRIST CURL ~ 35 × 12 - 2 sets
SET   (BB WRIST CURL   ~ 70 × 20 - 2 sets
       (GRIPPER   -   2 sets of 25

ROWING ERGOMETER - 1500 meters in 6 minutes

BRAIN   END   11:30 AM
   MIND GEAR PR-2   TOTAL SETS = 33
   PROGRAM 2 ~ 15 minutes TOTAL TIME = 90 MINUTES
                           TOTAL ABS = 560 REPS

155

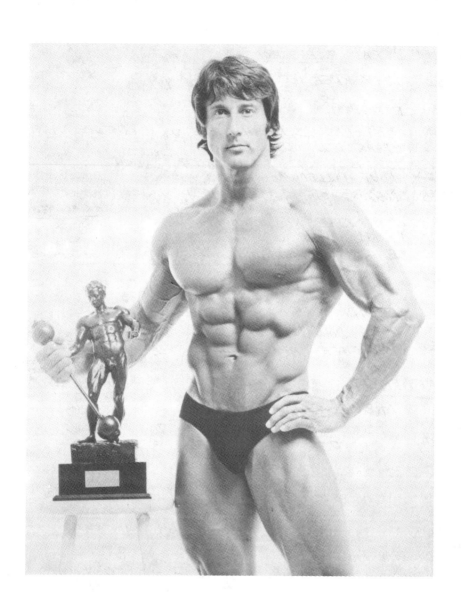

CHAPTER 8
SEASONAL TRAINING
FOR LONGEVITY

The solitary pine tree stands alone in the middle of an open field. Ages ago, there were other trees here but all of them have been gradually cut down. Every year when the woodcutters came, they surveyed the pine trees and selected the straightest ones to cut to provide lumber for houses and temples. No one paid the slightest attention to the solitary pine because it's trunk was so crooked and had sprouted so many side branches.

Hundreds of years have passed and the solitary pine has remained the only tree in the field. It provides homes for birds and squirrels and shade for weary travelers, but has often had to fight hurricanes all by itself. In the beginning, its roots would loosen and its branches would break. But its vitality of life anchored its roots so strongly that now they never loosen, and its branches are so tough that now they never break.

Its extra branches that have dried up provide more lumber than all the trees that formerly grew in the field. In the future, the solitary pine will be able to supply people with untold amounts of fuel and lumber, while remaining itself. This special uncompromising character that made it useless for good lumber also made the solitary pine what it is today. A character that cannot be lumber supplies more and better lumber. And this character also enables the pine to grow eternally. (1)

"The unfolding of the human potential from the present ordinary state of consciousness to the full extension of what is possible, has often been compared to the growth and flowering of a tree...Our roots are the heredity tendencies acquired from our ancestors; our trunk is the main axis of our life's growth through time; our branches are the traits, qualities, and abilities with which we extend and ramify ourselves; and our fruits are the products of our creativity, the seeds clothed in the nourishing flesh of our individual energies. These are the fruits of our actions by which we are known."

Ralph Mentzer (2)

"Man is the tree of life"   Deuteronomy, 20:19

"Woman is the image of the tree"   Paracelus

Human growth both physical and spiritual, emotional and intellectual develops throughout life much as the growth of a tree. And for every human endeavor involving this growth is a season where different trends and goals become evident. The maturing bodybuilder should take this fact of life into account and plan his/her training accordingly. All one need do is follow nature's example.

Mother nature divides a year into four seasons, each one distinct from the others: Winter is a time of conservation, hibernation, and inactivity; Spring, a time of rebirth, renewal, awakening, and new growth; Summer, of warmth, light, energy, and activity; Autumn, maturity, harvest, and Thanksgiving. A bodybuilder's year should be demarcated by seasons as well. Just as one season changes into another, a bodybuilder's goals should change as well. This has certainly been one of my own keys to training longevity.

Each of nature's seasons is 13 weeks--the time necessary to begin a new trend and follow it through to completion. I call these seasonal goals, "short-term goals", as contrasted to yearly goal which I refer to as "long-term goals". A complete year generates a completely new body. One season builds on the next, culminating in a physique that looks different, changed, improved.

The main element that distinguishes one season from another is length of daylight. Where I live, the sun is above the horizon on an average Winter day for about 10 hours, Spring 12 hours, Summer 14 hours, and Autumn 12 hours.

A graph of average sunlight hours for each season roughly resembles a graph of my training intensity:

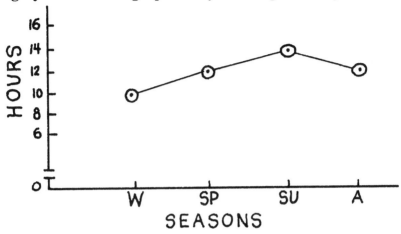

WINTER, for me, is off-season. I train every other day, specialize on weakpoints, and am not concerned about being extremely muscular or defined. I am content to allow a little more bodyfat, conserve energy, and concentrate on healing any injuries I might have incurred during the preceding harder training seasons I've just completed. Maintenance is the theme during Winter and the decreased time I spend training allows me to pursue other interests and activities. I work at balancing my lifestyle, devote more time to business, cultivating new relationships, and improving old ones.

Perhaps this change of training intensity is called "off season" or "post season" is related to sunshine. Research shows that decreasing amounts of sunlight during winter months affects moods, appetite, and can cause a form of depression known as seasonal affective disorder, or SAD (3). SAD is characterized by episodic bouts of depression combined with cravings for carbohydrate rich foods. These symptoms may sound familiar to Northern latitude city dwellers. Two distinct biochemical processes underlie these mood and appetite disorders. These systems involve the hormone melatonin which affects mood and subjective energy levels, and the neurotransmitter serotonin, which regulates appetite for carbohydrate rich foods.

Melatonin follows a circadian rhythm in humans and animals and is secreted by the pineal gland when it is dark, reaching its highest level in the middle of the night during sleep. The importance of the pineal gland is evidenced by the fact that it controls hibernation in some animals. Its parallel effect in humans seems to effect a desire to eat more and exercise less.

The pineal is the body's light meter which, along with the hypothalamus, functions to synchronize the body's metabolic processes in accordance with light from our environment. Recent studies indicate that the pineal gland may be a factor in longevity. Symptoms of aging may be cause by the progressive decline of melatonin synthesis in the pineal gland that occurs with age. (4)

Melatonin may also counteract the development of stress related disease. In humans, daytime melatonin levels are low and constant throughout life, but nighttime levels vary with age. The nighttime levels rise significantly up until age five and gradually decline throughout adulthood. Melatonin levels diminish greatly at about age 85. (5)

Also, since the weather is colder in Winter and we wear more clothing, we become less aware of what our bodies look like. I notice this trend beginning just after Thanksgiving, at the beginning of December. Unless I make a supreme effort, it seems that this big meal marks the start of the slowing down of metabolism and desire to exercise. Usually, I don't fight this natural tendency. After all, as I look back over the years past, I notice that I've been doing this for my whole bodybuilding career.

My training In Winter changes accordingly. If I am forced to take a layoff from training due to travel, illness, or injury, I try not to lay off for more than a week. My motivation for not wanting to stop all training for longer than a week is excessive soreness. I find that with a week layoff, my strength level stays pretty constant. My main loss during this short time out is the coordination or groove of the exercise movement. When I start back after a week off, I always reduce my exercise poundages by about 10 percent. This allows me to do my repetitions in perfect form.

For many people, a good possibility for post season training is to train the whole body each workout, two or three times a week. I almost never train this way myself, because I have too many favorite exercises for each bodypart and training the whole body would make my workout too long. A full body workout is just too much for me to confront in one training session. However, if you are a beginner, the full body workout is a good way to start because you don't have too many exercises to do. See Chapter 3 for the full body workout.

When I resume training after a layoff, I start back with the two-way split, working upper body one day and legs the next, with a little bit of aerobics and abdominal work at the end of each workout. See Chapter 4 for a detailed description of the two-way split routine. I train every other day, and for the first two weeks, I do only one set of 15 to 20 repetitions of each exercise with slightly lighter weights than before, stretching after each set.

If I am sore the day following each workout, I will stay with one set of each exercise but with a slightly heavier weight than the first workouts. As soon as the soreness subsides a little, I go to two sets of each exercise, doing 12 to 15 reps on the first set, stretching 15 seconds, adding weight, then doing 8 to 12 reps on the second set. My goals during Winter training are to conserve energy, get enough rest, and experiment with new exercises.

I usually continue this two-way split maintenance routine into the first or second week of January. By this time, the realization that a new year has begun has fully entered my awareness. It seems to take a few weeks into the new year before I always write the correct year when I date my checks. When I start getting the date right every time, I know it's time to move into the three-way split routine (see Chapter 6 for description of the 3 way split). I begin to train in a 6 day cycle as follows: Day 1-Back, biceps, forearms, abs, aerobics;

Day 2-Thighs, calves, abs, aerobics; Day 3-Rest; Day 4-Chest, shoulders, triceps, abs, aerobics; Day 5-Rest; Day 6-Rest. Repeat.

The 3-way split done in a 6 day cycle is a wonderful way to build strength and muscle. Each time you work a muscle group you work it hard and then give it plenty of rest to let it recuperate and grow. As a result, you are strong every workout and will make more rapid progression with weight increments. The 6 day cycle is much easier on my elbow and shoulder joints, since I always get two days rest between upper body workouts. I start my 6 day cycle with 2 sets of each exercise, my first set being 10 to 12 reps, and increasing the weight on my second set for 8 to 10 reps. I follow this scheme of sets and reps right up until the first day of Spring at which time I move up to 3 sets of each exercise. I begin using the weight star method described in Chapter 7 and my goals are to increase size and strength and improve muscular proportions.

SPRING is a time of rebirth for my muscles with getting back into good shape as its theme, and I now feel the need for more sunshine in my life coupled with the urge to train harder. Since light stimulates the pineal gland exclusively by way of the eyes, this may explain why sunlight and its seasonal variations can effect the way we feel. I really don't get the urge to begin intensified training until the spring, and as the weather gets warmer, I seem to get stronger. I'ts harder for me to get into top physical condition in the Winter. The sun keeps my muscles and joints warm and, providing I don't overdo exposure to the sun, makes me stronger in my workouts.

Sunbathing has always been a ritual with bodybuilders that enhances muscular definition. A suntan makes the skin feel tighter and enables the sunbather to lose excess water. I am very careful to acquire a suntan gradually and avoid burning. I apply Vaseline to my lips, knees, and lower legs to avoid dryness or chaffing, use moisturizer after sunbathing, and make sure to include enough oils like lecithin and olive oil in my diet.

In spite of all the research linking sun exposure to skin cancer, sunbathing still seems to be as popular as ever, especially with people on vacation who want to relax. "The only really clear thing", according to Dr. Jacob Liberman, "is that overexposure to the sun, in conjunction with certain skin types is a major factor in the development of skin cancer" (6). Liberman recommends that if you sunbathe for longer than one hour at a time, to work up gradually to it, avoiding exposure between 10am and 2pm when sun intensity is strongest.

Still, I feel it's best to get too little sun than to get too much sun. Being a little depressed is still better than having a little skin cancer or a lot of dry wrinkled skin. Parsimony always enables me to err on the conservative side. Just as I don't train every day, I don't sunbathe every day either. And I only intentionally seek sunshine between Spring and early Autumn. Your skin needs a rest too.

As a result of my rekindled desire to train harder, my Spring workouts become more intense since I am doing 3 sets of each exercise. Spreading my 3 way split routine over 6 days gives me enough time to rest and recuperate, keeps my enthusiasm high, and my strength keeps building. As a result, I am in really good shape by the first day of Summer.

SUMMER

In June I move up to the 5 day cycle using the 3 way split--training 2 days in a row, resting the third day, training the fourth day, and resting the fifth day. I continue to do 3 sets of each exercise but since I have one less day of rest, I make sure to conserve my energy so I don't get over-trained. If I'm feeling tired, I'll alternate a 5 day cycle with a 6 day cycle and pick up an extra rest day this way. I continue using the weight star method. My goals now are to build up my exercise poundages gradually and continue building size and strength without sacrificing shape and muscular definition in all bodyparts. I continue to train this way right up until the end of August.

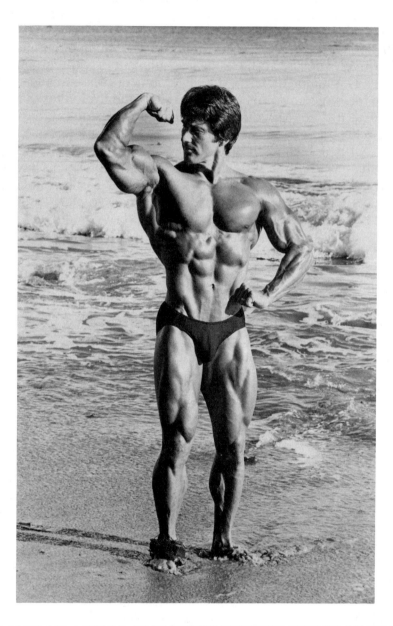

FRANK AT AGE 36, ONE WEEK BEFORE 1978 OLYMPIA

AUTUMN

I move up to the four day cycle, training three days in a row and resting the fourth day, using the advanced routine 3 way split (see Chapter 12) with 3 sets of each exercise during September and October. I begin using the time star method and as a result, I maximize my muscular definition and endurance and reach my long term goal for the year of peak physical condition. I do this every year even though I no longer enter bodybuilding competition. Getting in top condition is a great goal in itself, and these days I'm motivated out of a sense of curiosity to see just how good I can get.

After I reach my peak physical condition for the year, I begin to step down my training. I revert back to the 5 day cycle doing 2 sets of each exercise and do this right up until Thanksgiving. Then I move into maintenance as I described earlier. I never reach a sticking point and my progress is planned and deliberate. Since I'm not worried about being in top shape constantly, I have time to pursue other interests and activities in my life. My seasonal approach is a major factor accounting for my training longevity.

A SEASONAL APPROACH TO FAT LOSS GOALS

Since not everyone wants to build strength and muscle as I do, here is a seasonal progression which can be used by both men and women interested in losing bodyfat and toning muscles without building them:

December, January, February - Do the full body routine in Chapter 3, 3 days a week, 2 sets of each exercise, with a half hour of aerobics at the end of the workout. By the third week in January, move up to 3 sets of each exercise with 45 minutes of aerobics at end of workout. Goal- Keep bodyweight down by training quickly and aerobics, avoid binge eating over the holidays.

March, April, May - Do the 2 way split in Chapter 5, 4 days a week, 3 sets of each exercise, with 45 minutes of aerobics at the end of the workout. Use the time star method. Goal - Lose an average of one pound a week by keeping calories down and extra aerobics or ab-aerobics.

June, July, August - Do the 2 way split in Chapter 5, 5 days a week, 3 sets of each exercise, with 45 minutes of aerobics at end of workout. Continue with time star method. Goal - continue losing one pound a week.

September, October, November - Do the 2 way split in Chapter 5, 6 days a week, 3 sets of each exercise, with 45 minutes of aerobics at end of workout. Continue time star method. Goal - Continue to lose an average of one pound a week until desired bodyweight is attained; then increase caloric intake slightly.

RELATION BETWEEN AGE AND TRAINING CYCLES

Here is a summary of all the different ways I've trained over the years, and how I predict I'll train when I'm in my 60's. Parsimony has influenced my training as I've grown older. On the average, I now train less frequently but harder with more emphasis on deep relaxation between workouts. (2 day cycle means it takes me two days to work the entire body; 3 day cycle, 3 days to work the entire body, etc.):

Puberty through 20's - 2 day cycle, training 6 days a week on the 2 way split routine. In training for the Mr. America and Mr. Universe contests in 1968 when I was 26 years old, I made great progress training 2 days on, one day off up until the last month. Then I moved up to training 6 days a week. This is a tough schedule but the high energy of youth seems to allow for it.

30's - 3 day cycle training 6 days a week on the 3 way split routine. Actually, I trained this way from age 27 to age 37. This was the peak of my training career. I worked each bodypart twice a week, abdominals every day, and did a moderate amount of aerobic work.

40's - 4 day cycle: 3 days on, 1 day off, using the 3 way split routine. I began using this system in 1979 in my training for the Mr. Olympia. As a result of the extra rest day, I was able to gain additional size and strength. This is my favorite way to train when I want to get in top condition.

50's - 5 day cycle: 2 days on, one day off, one on, one off, using the 3 way split routine. This is an even better way to train for size and strength. I train this way most of the year now (except when I want to peak and use the 4 day cycle) and find I have more training enthusiasm when I train on the 5 day cycle, probably because I get more rest and can recuperate better from hard workouts.

60's - 6 day cycle: 2 days on, one day off, one on, two days off using the 3 way split routine. This routine gives me two days rest between upper body training days, allowing me to train heavy with enough time to heal. I often use the 6 day cycle now for maintenance since it allows me to keep using the same 3 way split routine: Day 1-Back, biceps, forearms; Day 2-Legs; Day 3-Chest, shoulders, triceps. Abdominal work and aerobics are done every training day.

70's and above - 7 day cycle: use the three way split and train three times a week (Monday, Wednesday, Friday or Tuesday, Thursday, Saturday). I sometimes use this program for maintenance or when I'm traveling.

At age 52 I find myself going back and forth between a 5, 6, and a 7 day cycle on the three way split and only using the 4 day cycle right before I want to peak. I am training less frequently but harder each workout and my enthusiasm is high.

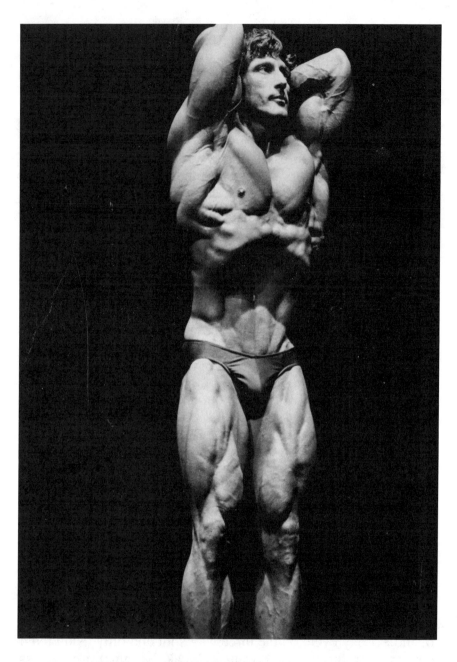

STOMACH VACUUM POSE, MR. OLYMPIA 1979

CHAPTER 9
ZANE NUTRITION

Once there was a man who had an enormously large stomach and ate everything in sight. One day he could find nothing to eat and, suffering so much, he sought help from a wise man who told him:

"Contemplate that your stomach is as empty as the sky. Let the fire burn as when you are hungry. Let all the visible world be edible and drinkable. And let it be consumed as you eat it."

The hungry man meditated with such devotion that the sun and moon hid themselves. So the wise man said, "you have eaten all the food; now meditate without it." So the hungry man did. The sun and moon reappeared and he realized the integration of appearances and emptiness. No longer hungry, the man attained great power, reduced his stomach, and inspired many people. (1)

Obesity is a challenge that confronts many aging people as their basal metabolism slows down. In my years of working with overweight clients, I've noticed one thing they all seem to have in common is "binge eating". Ingesting large amounts of high caloric junk food is how many people cope with stress. Whereas they may have gotten away with this when they were younger, this unchecked bad habit has now become out of control and has resulted in the middle age spread. Instead of dealing directly with the problem that is producing the stress, they unconsciously deal with their unpleasant emotions and pacify being fed up by eating to excess.

Reducing stress in this matter is called emotionally focused coping and is also a reason why people drink alcohol excessively. Drowning unpleasant emotions starts as a form of coping with stress and develops into a full blown habit. Moderate drinkers who consume one or two drinks a day claim it relaxes them and gives them pleasure, but as consumption escalates, a tolerance to alcohol develops and many of these people drink just to feel normal. The excess calories which are quickly ingested, play havoc with their blood sugar levels and metabolism and result in excess bodyfat. While alcohol in moderation improves beneficial cholesterol levels (HDL) and seems to stimulate the appetite especially for meat, alcoholic beverages should be avoided by those who desire to lose weight. The addictive nature of alcohol make it a substance that is easily abused.

Basal metabolism--the energy output required to keep heart, lungs, and brain functioning--slows with age. Men and women over 50 need at least 300 fewer daily calories than people in their early twenties to maintain the same bodyweight. Undernutrition without malnutrition can be the most important aspect of dietary modulation of lifespan. In such a regimen, the total intake of calories is limited but there is no lack of essential nutrients like amino acids, vitamins, minerals, and essential fatty acids (2). However, there's no need to starve yourself when you engage in a regular program of vigorous exercise. What's needed is a limited caloric intake that is nutritionally dense.

Recommended dietary allowance (RDA) charts tell us that a 154 pound man over 50 needs as many calories as a 7 to 10 year old 66 pound child, but 35% more protein than the child (3). So while caloric needs decrease with aging, protein needs increase. Protein deficiencies are common in the elderly, as many tend to eat a lot of refined carbohydrates devoid of substantial protein to meet the body's anabolic requirements for repair of muscle.

As we age, our hormonal production slows down. A goal of the aging bodybuilder is to maximize growth hormone (GH) secretion in as many natural ways as possible. In an experiment with elderly men by Dr. Daniel Rudman of the Medical College of Wisconsin (4), men treated with growth hormone showed and 8.8% increase in lean muscle mass, a 14.4% decrease in bodyfat, and a 7.1% increase in skin thickness. These men were given synthetic growth hormone injections several times a week for six months--a very costly program not without the risk of side effects. But the GH actually reversed the aging process by helping the men build muscle, increase skin thickness, and lose bodyfat. It makes sense, that to improve longevity means to maximize your own natural GH secretion in ways that are safe and affordable.

MAXIMIZE GH SECRETION

GH is secreted by the anterior pituitary gland in the brain. There are three ways to maximize this natural secretion:

1. **Weight-training** - Doing slow negative repetitions with enough weight so that you get a maximum pump in as short a time as possible. This is known as high intensity training.

2. **Slow wave sleep** - Since the brain secretes GH at the lowest delta brain wave frequency of slow wave sleep, duplicating delta wave frequencies with mind/body relaxation exercise (see Chapter 10) can assist in deep relaxation necessary for muscle growth and repair.

3. **Nutrition** - Cutting back on fat intake, eating substantial protein (1 gram per pound of desired bodyweight) and ingesting GH releasing amino acids between meals.

NUTRITIONAL MODULATION OF GH

Since we've already covered weight training in chapters 2 through 6 and will discuss low frequency brain wave entrainment in chapter 10, let's focus on how to enhance GH secretion nutritionally. The major variables are protein, carbohydrate, fat intake, and total calories.

Since we can calculate the percentage of calories eaten daily from fat, we can monitor fat loss. Since GH secretion is enhanced by a low fat diet, it makes sense to lower your fat intake. Some authorities say go as low as only 10 percent of total calories from dietary fat, but I personally feel best when my average daily fat intake is 20 to 25 percent. When I get under 15 percent my hunger increases, I lose energy, strength, and joint pain seems to increase. An adequate but not excessive fat intake alleviates these symptoms and gives me extra energy to train hard.

So **step 1** is to lower fat intake to somewhere between 25% and 15%. **Step 2** is to keep protein intake between 0.5 and 1 gram per pound of bodyweight and carbohydrates about 25% greater. Since I weigh 180 pounds, I eat an average of 180 grams of protein and 225 grams of carbohydrate daily. Since both protein and carbs contain 4 calories per gram: (180 + 225) x 4 = 1620 calories from these two macro-nutrient sources. My fats average about 38 grams per day, so 38 x 9 calories/gram = approx. 340 calories from fats. 1620 + 340 = 1980 total calories per day.

The percentage of calories from fat in my diet is calculated by dividing 340 by 1980, giving 17% of the calories in my diet come from fat. I notice that the lower this percentage gets, the less bodyfat I seem to carry. For me, getting in shape means eating approximately 10 calories for every pound of my bodyweight, keeping the percent of calories from fat under 25%, protein at least 180 grams, and carbs up to 225 grams on an average day.

This amount of protein is necessary to build muscle and I get it from both animal and vegetable sources. Eating a wide variety of protein foods in moderation will insure that you get a balanced allocation of amino acids, vitamins, and minerals. I also find 160 to 225 grams of carbohydrate eaten predominantly earlier in the day gives me enough energy to train hard and stay alert. Eating more carbohydrates than you need for immediate energy purposes results in storing this extra energy as glycogen as well as fat for future energy purposes. Nutrients get partitioned after exercise less toward fat storage and more toward nourishing muscle tissue. However, this doesn't mean that you should eat large high caloric meals after a late evening workout if you are trying to lose bodyfat.

Perhaps the most scientific way to determine your optimum carbohydrate intake is to use "keto stix" to measure the amount of carbs necessary to keep you just slightly out of ketosis. Ketosis occurs when your carbs are low and your body begins to convert stored bodyfat into free fatty acids in your bloodstream to be burned for energy. This process is called lipolysis and is indicated by urinating on a keto stix. If it turns from biege to purple this means you are in ketosis. If the keto stix turns dark purple this means you are in heavy ketosis and are probably burning protein from muscle tissue as well as stored bodyfat. I used keto stix when I competed and found the best range was very light purple for losing bodyfat only.

Drinking an adequate amount of liquids during the day is important to prevent dehydration. If your urine is very yellow you should drink more water. Coffee, tea, and alcohol are all dehydrating, and so is too high a level of protein without adequate carbohydrate. Carbs are like sponges that hold fluid in the muscle. A person who eats very high carbs in relation to protein will tend to fluctuate more in bodyweight due to fluid retention. Competitive bodybuilders generally avoid sugar as well as salt prior to a competition as both retain fluids in the body.

As you get older, your sensation of thirst becomes a less reliable gauge for how much fluid you should drink during the day, so be sure to drink at least two liters of fluid daily. My favorite fluids are water, carbonated or sparkling water, herbal teas, and coffee in moderation. Occasionally I drink some low sodium caffein free diet sodas. I usually make it a point not to drink calories as are found in fruit juices. The concentrated sugar in fruit juices is rapidly released in the bloodstream causing a large amount of insulin secretion. It's much better to eat fruit than to drink its juice because the fruit fiber provides a gradual release of the naturally occuring sugar in the fruit.

The **third step** in nutritional modulation of GH release is to take growth hormone releasing amino acids either right before meals and begin your meal with the carbohydrate portion--or take the GH releasers between meals with a small portion of carbohydrate (the insulin secreted by the pancreas when carbs are eaten helps the amino acids absorb into the cells of the body). I call this method "amino acid snacking" as it is a good way to add the ultimate effects of extra protein to your diet without adding fat. Vitamins and minerals should also be taken right afterward as they assist in amino acid absorption.

I use a very high grade of free form amino acids (intravenous pharmaceutical grade) in capsule form which contain the branched chain amino acids L-Leucine, L-Isoleucine, L-Valine, plus the GH releasing amino acids L-Glycine, L-Tyrosine, L-Methionine, L-Arginine, L-Lysine, and L-Phenylalanine. The capsules also contain L-Histidine and L-Threonine and are contained in a packet and give me a total of 2100 mg. of amino acids in free form per packet.

Also contained in this packet are the following **VITAMINS**: Vitamin A - 8000 IU, Vitamin C - 100 mg, B-1 - 65 mg, B-2 - 45 mg, Niacin - 20 mg., Niacinamide - 75 mg, Calcium Pantothenate - 325 mg, B-6 - 110 mg, Pyridoxal 5' Phosphate - 4.5 mg, B-12 - 420 mcg, Folic Acid - 360 mcg, Biotin - 420 mcg, PABA - 90 mg, Vitamin E - 120 IU, Choline Bitartrate - 125 mg, Inositol - 50 mg; and **MINERALS**: Calcium - 80 mg, Magnesium - 50 mg, Potassium - 39 mg, Manganese - 6 mg, Zinc - 12 mg, Copper - 60 mcg, Selenium - 40 mcg, Molybdenum - 60 mcg, Chromium - 60 mcg, Iron - 7.2 mg, Iodine - 30 mcg. Taking amino acids, vitamins, and minerals in this packeted format makes supplementation to the diet very convenient.

When in hard training, I take 1/2 teasp. of L-Tyrosine in powdered form in the morning before my workout to increase alertness (it is a precursor to hormones such as thyroxin and adrenalin), gives me more energy (since L-tyrosine is needed to make the neurotransmitter dopamine in the brain), a half tsp. L-Glutamine sublingually to increase alertness and spare glucose for energy and build reserves in muscles, as well as L-Proline to help rebuild collagen in connective tissues. For a complete description of the exact function of each vitamin, mineral, and amino acid, see *Zane Nutrition* (5).

Supplementing the diet is a good idea if you want to get the most nutritional value from your eating. I recommend using a computer program to keep track of the foods you eat during the day. Of course you can do this without a computer if you don't have one by using *Zane Nutrition* as your guide. To really go in depth I suggest the *Corinne Netzer Encyclopedia of Food Values* (6). One thing I noticed from keeping track of the foods I eat, was that there were certain nutrients I wasn't getting enough of in my normal daily eating pattern, especially Vitamin B-12, zinc, folic acid, and magnesium. This is the problem with diets that lack certain foods: cut out egg yolks and lose the sulfur bearing amino acids L-Methionine and L-Cystiene necessary for good hair, skin, and GH release; eliminate dairy products and calcium and the amino acid L-Tryptophan diminish; stop eating red meat and watch your iron, B-12, and zinc intake go down. It's best not to eliminate any food entirely. Supplementing your diet with vitamins, minerals, enzymes, and amino acids is good nutritional insurance.

Some other good supplements to take with meals are liver extract, essential fatty acids derived from germ oil concentrates, and lecithin. These nutrients provide energy, keep the skin and hair healthy, and cut down on appetite for fatty foods. Also pancreatin digestive enzymes with meals can help you build muscle by helping you better digest your food.

NUTRITION AND ANABOLIC STEROIDS

It seems that every seminar I teach, the question of steroid usage comes up. With more and more people entering bodybuilding, the competition for titles is tougher than ever before. It seems that the bodybuilders getting the majority of publicity are those who have used steroids to develop maximum size, strength, and muscularity. As a result, the bodybuilding public has come to expect massive Herculean muscles from its champions.

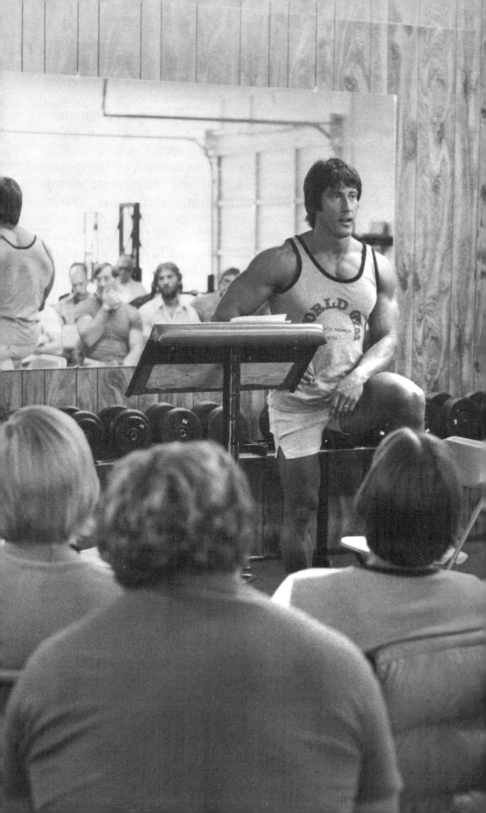

Those who have used steroids will tell you that they have made gains in strength and muscular bodyweight in relatively short periods of time as compared to when they were not using these drugs. As they begin to depend on them for their muscle size and strength gains, these bodybuilders never learn how to make any real progress without steroids.

When used under medical supervision, anabolic steroids were shown to have been effective in increasing protein synthesis, strength, bodyweight, and hemoglobin in anemia; useful in treating anorexia, senility, postmenopausal osteoporosis, pituitary dwarfism, burns, gastrointestinal disease; and recommended for pre- and post- operative care-- the original purpose for which they were intended--supportive treatment for acute and chronic illness, and tonic action in the elderly.

On the negative side, anabolic steroids, if used excessively and indiscriminately without medical supervision, can cause prostrate and breast cancer, benign prostrate hypertrophy, cardiac disease, kidney disease, liver disease, edema or abnormal water retention and swelling, abnormal bone development in children and adolescents, nausea, vomiting, diarrhea, excitation and hypertension, insomnia, chills, changes in libido, acne, high blood pressure, jaundice, hepatitis, inhibition of testicular function, impotence, male pattern baldness, and gynecomastia (or "bitch tits") in men, and voice deepening, increased amount of facial hair, clittoral enlargement, and menstrual irregularities and depression in women (7).

Another problem associated with steroid use is addiction. While it is generally agreed that steroids are non-addictive, the strength and muscle building effects associated with steroid usage has enticed many bodybuilders to keep using the drugs without going off them long enough. Tests have shown a prolonged impairment of testicular endocrine function resulting in loss of sex drive after athletes stopped using steroids (8). So rather than experience the depression, lack of sexual drive, and loss of strength accompanying steroid cessation, many strength athletes stay on these drugs for prolonged periods of time or alternate their use with other anabolic steroids or testosterone escalating drugs. This is very dangerous and can lead to uncontrollable aggression, depression and permanent personality changes in addition to the potential damage to the body.

Bodybuilding is a lifetime commitment and young competitors shouldn't be so impatient to make it to the top. When I see massive muscular bodybuilders winning high level competitions with only a few years of training it makes me wonder just how long their bodybuilding careers will last. Judging standards need to be changed so that excessive size and muscular density are not overemphasized. The metaphors associated with such over-development aptly describe the mental state associated with size obsession--thickness and density are not synonyms for intelligence!

A really well developed body takes many years to build and physical qualities like symmetry, proportion, and definition have little to do with steroid use and more to do with intelligent training. Bodies built with steroids look mass produced and lack individuality because they are built in too short a period of time. Steroids are definitely part of the bodybuilding as character armor syndrome. There is no art involved in mass production.

While education and enlightenment about the dangers of steroids are certainly helpful and necessary, what's really needed is a safe substitute for anabolic steroids that is just as effective when it comes to building strength and muscle, but without the dangerous side effects. Medical science has given us steroids, now hopefully it will discover something healthier and better. A safe effective magical pill would certainly make a lot of athletes very happy.

In the final analysis, what substances people use or abuse is a matter of personal responsibility. Instead of resorting to steroids, people should consider the common sense alternatives which are currently available. One avenue to making gains without resorting to steroids is to maximize the anabolic variable of the bodybuilding equation: Rest--the deep relaxation techniques associated with GH release are totally neglected by bodybuilders (see Chapter 10), and nutritional supplementation to an already healthy diet.

According to hormone replacement specialist Edmund Chein MD of Palm Springs, California, building muscle past age 40 is difficult unless your thyroid, testosterone, and growth hormone levels are those of a healthy person in his early twenties. Dr. Chein suggests making hormonal levels adequate if one expects to build maximum muscle mass. Against anabolic steroids, he has helped steroid addicted individuals.

Supplementing the diet with adequate amounts of vitamins, minerals, essential fatty acids, Creatine Monohydrate, Liver Extract, and enzymes along with the free form amino acids which are linked to natural GH production in the body, such as L-Tyrosine, L-Glutamine, L-Methionine, and Glycine, as well as the branched chain amino acids L-Leucine, L-Isoleucine, and L-Valine can be helpful in facilitating muscle growth. Amino acids are the building blocks of protein and muscle tissue as well as precursors for hormones (human growth hormone is composed of 191 amino acids bonded together in a specific order) and neuro-transmitters which effect metabolism and behavior.

Isn't it possible that these substances might be used in place of steroids without risking the dangerous side effects? It may take longer, but it is infinitely safer and legal. Dietary supplements, however, do not justify a poor diet. They work best when you are eating highly nutritious foods.

MY DAILY EATING PATTERN

Breakfast usually consists of cooked grains like oats, rye, triticale, barley, or oat groats served with fresh or frozen berries and a banana. I like to have this breakfast two or three hours before my workout as it is loaded with complex carbohydrates. I take my supplements immediately before I start eating and usually have 6 ounces of freshly brewed coffee as I finish. Coffee in moderation has been shown to be an ergogenic aid which promotes the burning of bodyfat for energy, a stimulant which enhances muscle contraction, a laxative, and has recently been shown to increase HDL levels in men who drank two cups a day by researchers at John Hopkins Medical Institution in Baltimore. So if you drink coffee, be sure not to have more than two cups a day, and never on an empty stomach.

Another breakfast which I eat on alternate days, provides more protein, less carbohydrate and digests more quickly, is two or three soft boiled eggs with two slices of whole grain toast. Those concerned about the cholesterol content of egg yolks should be aware that stress is a much more potent contributor to high serum cholesterol levels than dietary fat intake. Results of a study of the effects of job stress on serum cholesterol (9) showed subject's cholesterol levels to be 17% higher during high stress periods as compared to low stress periods. Diet was not systematically related to cholesterol. Compared to investigations of dietary effects of cholesterol, a 70% increase in cholesterol intake would be required to match the fluctuations in serum cholesterol caused by stress (10).

My lunch and dinner are combinations of some kind of meat and vegetables. I may eat starches (pasta, bread, baked yam or potato, brown rice) for lunch but never for dinner. It's best to eat starches earlier in the day so they can supply you with energy throughout your waking hours. Eating a starchy meal late in the day forces your body to store the excess energy as fat and glycogen. This can increase your bodyfat stores unless you train hard after this late meal.

Lunch is usually a high protein meal with vegetables, and dinner is a lower calorie meal with low carbohydrate vegetables and meat, poultry, or fish. Eating a light dinner early--never after 7 pm--is perhaps the most important part of losing excess bodyfat.

Speaking of fat, any fat you eat is first stored in and on your body before it can be used for energy. So I don't eat pure fats like butter and cream--instead, I keep my fat intake low by eating them as they naturally occur with protein and carbohydrates.

In summary, my carbohydrate intake is greatest for breakfast, lesser for lunch, and least for dinner. Protein is moderate for breakfast, high for lunch, and moderate for dinner. Fats are low for all three meals. Eating this way has enabled me to have enough energy for hard workouts, enough protein for repairing exercised muscle, and just enough fats for healthy skin, hair, health and integrity of internal organs, and prevention of excessive hunger as well as adding taste to my meals.

MY 4 DAY EATING CYCLE

Here is a sample of our typical way of eating in a 4 day cycle. My wife Christine follows the restricted calorie version while I follow the regular version. This allows us the convenience of preparing the same meals since we eat different proportions of some of the foods.

DAY 1

Upon arising: Free form amino acids, vitamins, minerals.

Breakfast: 1/3 cup long grain rye, 1/3 oat groats or steel cut oats, 1/3 cup mueseli. I bring the rye to a boil in 12 ounces of water, turn off the heat, add the oat groats and soak overnight. In the morning I bring the mixture to a boil, add the mueseli, cook 5 minutes, and let stand with lid on. Add fresh or frozen berries, and one fresh sliced banana, and sweetened with fructose (2tsp.) or honey (2tbsp). I sip one cup of black freshly ground filtered coffee toward the end of the meal.

Lunch: Chicken frajita (8 oz chicken, 1/4 head shredded lettuce, 1 tomato, 1 tbsp. salsa, 2 corn tortillas.) glass of water and supplements.

Dinner: 2 handfulls of fresh salad mixture, diet ranch dressing, 1 oz shredded Swiss cheese, 8 oz broiled filet mignon. Supplements taken with 8 oz caffein free Diet Coke.

Snack: 1 medium fresh pear.

DAILY TOTALS:
CALORIES 1560, PROTEIN 145 GRAMS, CARBS 160 GRAMS, FAT 38 GRAMS, 22% CALORIES FROM FAT.

RESTRICTED CALORIE VERSION: Eliminate 1/3 cup of oat groats or steel cut oats and sweeten with Equal or Sweet & Low instead of fructose or honey for breakfast. Reduce chicken to 4 oz. and drop one tortilla for lunch, and eliminate the cheese and drop to 4 oz filet mignon for dinner. This reduces DAILY TOTALS to:

CALORIES 960, PROTEIN 75 GRAMS, CARBS 120 GRAMS, FAT 20 GRAMS, WITH 19% CALORIES FROM FAT.

DAY 2
Upon arising: Amino acids, vitamins, minerals.

Breakfast: 1/2 fresh grapefruit sweetened with Equal, 2 slices whole grain toast, 2 soft boiled eggs, supplements with water, 8 oz coffee after meal.

Lunch: green salad with oil and vinegar, 2 olives, 1/2 tomato; spaghetti, mushrooms, garlic, light olive oil, Parmesan cheese, 1 slice French bread; water and supplements.

Dinner: one can (6 & 1/8 oz) water packed tuna, 1 tbsp low fat mayonaisse, alfalfa sprouts, 1/2 apple, supplements with 8 oz diet root beer.

Snack: 1 medium fresh peach

DAILY TOTALS:
CALORIES 1640, PROTEIN 115 GRAMS, CARBS 195 GRAMS, FAT 44 GRAMS, 24% OF CALORIES FROM FAT.

RESTRICTED CALORIE VERSION: drop 1 egg for breakfast, Eliminate olives, olive oil, and Parmesan cheese, drop to 4 oz pasta for lunch. Reduce to 3 oz of tuna and 1 teaspoon low fat mayonaisse for dinner. This reduces DAILY TOTALS TO:

CALORIES 1340, PROTEIN 85 GRAMS, CARBS 180 GRAMS, FAT 30 GRAMS, WITH 20% OF CALORIES FROM FAT.

DAY 3
Upon arising: amino acids, vitamins, minerals

Breakfast: Oats and rye (soak rye overnight, then add oats after bringing to a boil, boil 5 minutes, sit for 5 minutes with lid on); Mixed with frozen berries and sliced banana, sweetened with honey. 8 oz coffee after meal.

Lunch: two medium turkey drumsticks, one medium baked yam, peppermint tea with equal, supplements with water.

Dinner: Green salad with diet ranch dressing, 6 oz Filet Mignon broiled rare, 8 oz Caffein Free Diet Coke with supplements.

Snack: 1 medium fresh apple.

DAILY TOTALS:
CALORIES 1460, PROTEIN 125 GRAMS, CARBS 190 GRAMS, FAT 22 GRAMS, 14% OF CALORIES FROM FAT.

RESTRICTED CALORIE VERSION: use 1/4 cup each of oats and rye, eliminate banana, substitute equal for honey for breakfast. Drop one drumstick or substitute turkey breast for lunch. Reduce to 3 oz of lean steak for dinner.

DAILY TOTALS: CALORIES 950, PROTEIN 55 GRAMS, CARBS 160 GRAMS, FAT 10 GRAMS, 10% CALORIES FROM FAT.

DAY 4

Upon arising: Amino acids, vitamins, minerals

Breakfast: Swiss cheese omlette with one whole egg and two egg whites and one ounce of Swiss cheese. Baked potato (micro wave potato 8 to 10 minutes, wrap and let sit in aluminum foil 20 minutes). Peppermint/ephedra tea with equal, supplements with water.

Lunch: 12 oz chicken slow cooked in crock pot, steamed broccoli, carrots, and celery. Caffein Free Diet Coke with supplements.

Dinner: Seafood salad (shrimp, scallops, swordfish, lettuce, tomatoes, asparagus, red cabbage, cucumber, diet thousand island dressing. Sparkling mineral water with supplements.

Snack: 1 fresh medium orange

DAILY TOTALS:
CALORIES 1800, PROTEIN 180 GRAMS, CARBS 163 GRAMS, FAT 48 GRAMS, 24% CALORIES FROM FAT.

RESTRICTED CALORIE VERSION: Eat a smaller baked potato for breakfast and reduce to 4 oz chicken for lunch.

DAILY TOTALS: CALORIES 1250, PROTEIN 110 GRAMS, CARBS 135 GRAMS, FAT 30 GRAMS, 22% CALORIES FROM FAT.

4 DAY AVERAGE:
CALORIES 1615, PROTEIN 141 GRAMS, CARBS 177 GRAMS, FAT 38 GRAMS, 21% CALORIES FROM FAT.

4 DAY RESTRICTED CALORIE VERSION AVERAGE:
CALORIES 1125, PROTEIN 81 GRAMS, CARBS 150 GRAMS, FAT 22 GRAMS, 18% CALORIES FROM FAT.

MY DIET FOR MUSCULAR GROWTH

Several months after my 52nd birthday I began experimenting with a special diet which enabled me to add 10 pounds of muscular bodyweight in under 8 weeks!

Upon Arising - Amino acids, vitamin- mineral packet with carbonated water.

Breakfast - Two cups fresh or sugar free frozen strawberries (thawed in micro-wave oven), 10 oz. low sodium diet soda, one medium sliced bananna, 1 teaspoon psyllium (sugar free "Metamucil"), two packets of **METAFORM** (11) original flavor which supplied 720 calories, 74 grams protein, 100 grams carbohydrate, and 4 grams fat). I mixed these ingredients into a thick pudding and ate it slowly with a spoon while I sipped 8 oz decaffinated coffee and swallowed 5 liver extract capsules, 4 pancreatic enzyme tablets, 2 lecithin/Essential Fatty Acid capsules, and one mineral capsule with water.

Workout 3 hours after breakfast

15 minutes before lunch - Amino acids, vitamin-mineral packet with carbonated water.

Lunch - 14 ounces 93% lean ground sirloin broiled with low fat/low sodium swiss cheese on top with two whole wheat crackers, 4 liver extract capsules, 2 lecithin/EFA capsules, 2 pancreatic enzyme capsules, one mineral capsule, with low sodium sparkling mineral water.

Afternoon snack - One packet of **METAFORM** mixed in blender with one can of Diet Rite strawberry soda, with 3 liver extract capsules, 2 lecithin/EFA capsules, 2 pancreatic digestive enzyme capsules.

Aerobic/abdominal workout 2 hours later

15 minutes before dinner - Amino acids, vitamin-mineral packet with carbonated water.

Dinner - 8 ounces chicken breast (no skin) or fish, low carbohydrate steamed vegetable (such as asparagus, broccoli, zucchini, summer squash) or raw tomato, lettuce, alfafa sprouts; 2 liver capsules, 1 lecithin/EFA capsule, 2 pancreatic enzyme tablets, 1 mineral capsule, with Caffein Free Diet Coke.

Evening snack - Same **METAFORM** meal as breakfast but with chocolate flavor and no bananna.

DAILY TOTALS: 2740 calories, 310 grams protein, 240 grams carbohydrate, 60 grams fat, 19.7 % calories from fat.

My daily protein intake now averaged more than it had in the last ten years (pancreatin helped digest all this protein), and as a result I gained solid muscular bodyweight in a relatively short period of time. The great taste of the **METAFORM** enabled me to look forward to these high protein low fat meals and eliminated any cravings for sweets or fatty foods.

Here are some additional quickly prepared, low fat/high protein meals I eat when I don't feel like cooking:

My favorite soup recipe is 1 can of Health Valley non-fat Italian minestrone soup mixed with one 7 oz. can of water packed tuna (drain off water first). Cover bowl with plastic wrap and microwave for a little under 3 minutes. Add 1 slice of low fat/low sodium Swiss cheese (I use Swiss Alpine Lace) and 1 whole grain cracker. The quickly prepared meal gives 60 grams of protein and 30 grams of carbohydrate and very little fat. Another soup combination is Health Valley country corn and vegetable with 6 oz. sliced turkey breast which adds up to about the same amount of protein and carbs.

A good sandwich puts two whole grain crackers (10 grams of carbs) with 5 ounces of turkey breast and a slice of cheese (42 grams of protein) with lettuce, tomato, and/or sprouts. This gives 42 grams of protein and 12 grams of carbohydrate. Add lots of lettuce and/or spinach, crush the crackers and shred the turkey and cheese, add a low fat dressisng of your choice (I like Kraft fat free mayonnaise) and you have **a good salad**.

For more recipes see *THE COOKBOOK: A COMPANION TO ZANE NUTRITION* (12).

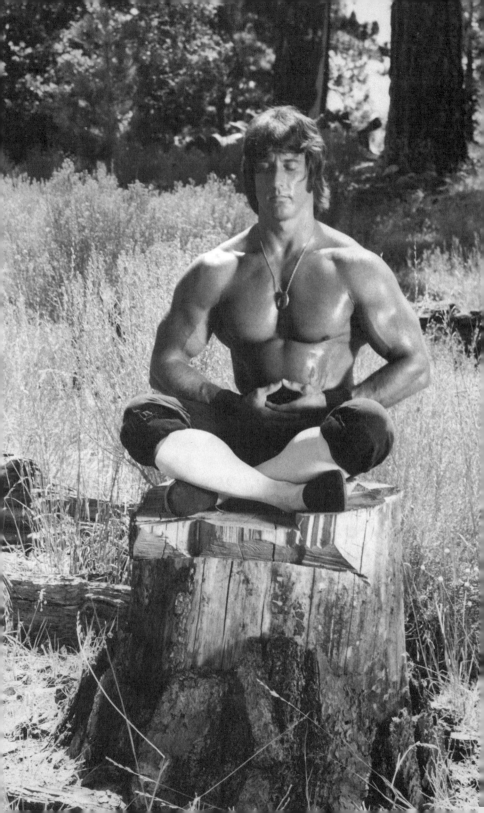

CHAPTER 10:
MIND/BODY EXCELLENCE

"Suppose we get several old-fashioned pendulum type grandfather clocks. Let us hang them on a wall and arrange their pendulums so that they will start out beating each at different angles, that is, out of phase with each other. In a day or two, we shall find that all the pendulums are beating in phase, as if locked together. (Pendulum length should be the same for all of them.) Here we see that the tiny amount of energy that was transmitted through the wall from clock to clock was sufficient to bring them into phase with each other. If we disturb one of the clocks, it will get locked into rhythm quite fast. The larger the number of oscillators (or objects that vibrate) within such a system, the more stable the system, and the more difficult it is to disturb. It will force a wayward oscillator back into line very quickly."

Itzhak Bentov (1)

"Unlike the fight-or-flight response, which is repeatedly brought forth in response to our difficult everyday situations and is elicited without conscious effort, the Relaxation Response can be evoked only if time is set aside and a conscious effort is made. Our society has given very little attention to the importance of relaxation...We could all greatly benefit by the re-incorporation of the Relaxation Response into our lives. At the present time, most of us are simply not making use of this remarkable innate, neglected asset."

Herbert Benson, M.D. (2)

Exercise is not all there is to bodybuilding. When we train we are not building the body, we are actually destroying it! Intensive exercise induces a condition which might be called "micro-trauma". Muscles heat up, small capillaries burst, and waste products such as lactic acid accumulate.

Without proper rest, deep relaxation, and good nutrition, our training efforts can result in a catabolic catastrophe.

Exercise is stress, since it is catabolic or destructive metabolism. A good form of stress, but stress nevertheless. Hans Selye defines stress as the rate of all the wear and tear on the body caused by life: "Stress is not even necessarily bad for you; it is also the spice of life, for any emotion, any activity causes stress. But, of course your system should be prepared to take it. The same stress which makes one person sick can be an invigorating activity for another" (3). Such is the case with bodybuilding, since everyone has a different threshold for the amount and intensity of training they can handle.

Stress management is important, because with age, autonomic nervous system (ANS) stereotypy increases. This means that we tend to respond the same way physiologically to stress as we grow older. ANS stereotypy is greatest between the ages of 40 through 59, making this middle segment of life a very susceptible period for the possible incidence of stress related disorders (4). These results may explain the increased incidence of health problems as people age. If this stereotyped response is frequently triggered by the environment, the person stays in a chronic fight-or-flight response, which eventually leads to homeostatic failure and illness.

We inherited the fight-or-flight response as part of our evolution. Although it is useful in emergency situations, we seldom have to do battle or run away to save our lives in today's society. Chronic unmanaged stress levels and the corresponding elicitation of the fight-or-flight response can lead to a permanent state of hypertension and high blood pressure (5).

I often ask people if they practice any form of stress management. They usually respond, "Yes, I exercise in the gym several times a week". While this does make them feel better, it is not true stress management. Stress management is anabolic, or constructive metabolism. It involves deep relaxation and comes in two forms:

THE TWO FORMS OF DEEP RELAXATION

1. Learning and eliciting the "Relaxation Response" during one's waking hours.

2. Getting enough deep restful sleep.

THE RELAXATION RESPONSE

In the early 1970's Dr. Herbert Benson of Harvard University coined the term "Relaxation Response" to describe the effects which occurred in practitioners of Transcendental Meditation. Unlike the fight-or-flight response which occurs automatically during emergencies, the Relaxation Response must be learned and practiced.

Meditation is a very simple technique which can evoke the Relaxation Response after enough skill is gained through practice. Physically, you need nothing to practice meditation except a quiet environment and a comfortable position. Meditation begins with concentration--the practice of focusing the mind on an object or stimulus. It is much like aiming an arrow at the center of a target. At first, the beginning archer shoots arrows all over the place, but with practice, he begins to group them in the center of the target. This aim is concentration and it involves a narrowing down of attention to exclude everything else but one's goal--the center. Concentration leads to one-pointedness--becoming centered.

Meditation is prolonged concentration, an unbroken flow of thought toward an object. It involves a continuous recycling of the stimulus or object of concentration through consciousness. But since our concentration isn't perfect, our

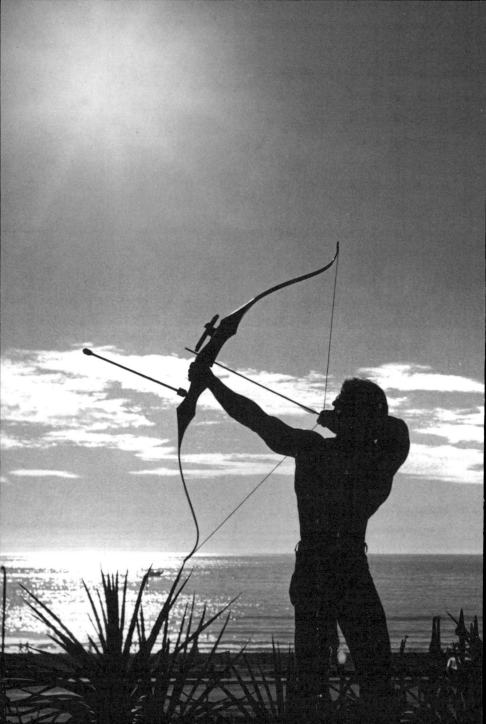

attention wanders. True meditation involves not only paying attention to the stimulus which is the object of our concentration, but also remembering to continue to generate and recycle the stimulus for the duration of the meditation session.

Probably the two most popular methods of meditation are Zen and Transcendental Meditation (TM). The beginning Zen meditation is called breath counting and involves simply counting each time you exhale up to the tenth exhalation, then starting over at one again. In the process of doing this, the mind wanders, you lose count or count past ten, and begin at one again. With practice, your concentration sharpens, your mind wanders less, and you begin to experience the Relaxation Response. A wonderful exposition of Zen Meditation is contained in Phillip Kapaleau's *Three Pillars of Zen*.

TM involves sitting relaxed in a quiet setting and repeating a "Mantram" or affirmation (see Chapter 7 for a list of such power phrases) over and over again. If you do this aloud it is called chanting, which is especially powerful when done with a group of people. The affirmation is any short statement which has a positive connotation for you. Repeating your affirmation is something you can do while engaging in activities that don't require your complete attention, like driving a car, walking, or doing abdominal exercises, or riding a stationary bicycle. By taking 20 minutes time out during the day and meditating, your affirmation will pop back into your mind at different times during the day along with its associated feeling of relaxation. Instead of letting your mind wander aimlessly, you can remove negativity and develop great mental and emotional power by focusing on positive affirmation.

Such positive affirmation played a central role in helping me win the Mr. Olympia Title three years in a row. I made a promise to myself to repeat my affirmation one million times a year during 1977, 78, and 79. My practice was especially intensive in the last weeks preceding competition with the result that negative thoughts never crossed my mind since my mind space was filled by positive affirmation. I became completely confident in my ability to win and learned the true meaning of having faith in myself. To me, faith came to mean certainty, or the absence of doubt.

People who take a course in TM are given a mantram, and while it's always helpful to have a teacher if you want to be successful in continuing to meditate, you can select your own affirmation by reading books on the subject. Two books I found helpful are John Blofeld's *Mantras*, and Eknath Earswaran's *Formulas for Transformation*. I knew when I found the affirmation that worked for me and I'll bet that you will too. The mantram I used for Mr. Olympia and still do is **"namu amida butsu"** which to me says thank you to the universe for creating my best possible future.

THE FITNESS BENEFITS OF MEDITATION

Although meditation has been practiced for thousands of years, scientific investigation expanded its perspecitve over the last few decades. Meditation can develop mastery of the mind/body connnection. With this mastery, one can achieve a higher level of fitness and a greater physique. It also can heighten perception of internal and external events, improve motor skill and reaction time, improve concentration and attention span, increase empathy and pleasure, improve memory and intelligence, enhance dream recall, alter body image, and increase energy and other fitness benefits (6,7,8,9).

My own experience with meditation confirms these research conclusions. I find that after a 15 minute meditation I'm able to concentrate more effectively on each exercise and get more from my workout in less time. The measure of a good workout is not how long you train but how intense you train: Get the most work done in the least amount of time.

My nutrition also benefits from the greater mind/body mastery that I develop as a result of meditation. I find myself desiring to eat foods most conducive to getting in great shape, enjoying these meals throughout the day. Many diets fail because they are based on deprivation which develops an unsatisfactory mind/body state. Because meditation builds a sense of inner peace, I get a great deal of pleasure from the taste of the foods I eat, and grow stronger. Meditation also helps me get the most from my post-workout recuperation. Much attention is given to maximizing workout performance, but not enough awareness is focused on the recuperation process. Hard workouts stimulate the muscles by tearing them down--muscles actually grow when you rest them. Putting all your effort into working out but ignoring recuperation is like investing your time and money destroying the building you own, but then forgetting to clear away the rubble and begin reconstruction! Instead you live in the ruins. After a workout, I revitalize by meditating.

PSYCHOLOGICAL BENEFITS OF MEDITATION

There also tremendous psychological benefits which accrue from the regular practice of meditation. Psychologist Daniel Goleman writes that meditation will: result in positive behavior change, reduce anxiety, improve self concept, increase energy, cause deep level personality changes toward mental health, improve musculature and posture, and boost resistance to pressure (10). In describing the *Abhidharma*, an Eastern psychological model of mental health, Goleman says:

"The basic unit of analysis in this model is a single moment of mind in succession of such moments in the stream of awareness. Each such moment is seen to be characterized by different flavors called mental factors. Those states that are unhealthy or unwholesome are those that are not conducive to calm, to tranquility, to equilibrium, to meditation, to the attainment of enlightenment.
The primary unhealthy mental factor is delusion or ignorance, a perceptual element defined as a cloudiness of mind that leads to misperception, confusion, and bewilderment. Delusion keeps us from seeing things clearly. It is the fundamental root of suffering. From a Western psychological

point of view, we would say that it is defended perception, as opposed to perception that does not need to hide anything from itself, which has no fear.

The second unhealthy factor is attachment, or clinging. The flavor of it is a selfish longing to satisfy desire, which exaggerates the attractiveness of that which is desired. It is a desire that distorts. It speaks to an addictive quality of longing. Clinging is selfish, love is not.

The third is anger, hostility, or ill will, an intense aversion that distorts reality too, but in the opposite direction from clinging. It makes us see things in a disagreeable light. It bewilders, deludes, and disturbs the mind.

The fourth is self-importance, or conceit, an inflated or superior self image that makes us, to quote one source, envious of superiors, competitive with equals and arrogant toward inferiors.

Another unwholesome factor is wrong view, the misapprehension or misdiscernment of things. having misperceived because of ignorance, you continue to misconstrue...We are talking about a fundamental perceptual distortion that then, in the flow of information, leads to miscategorizations, and to emotional reactions tied to those miscategorizations.

Another key addictive factor is indecisiveness, or perplexity, the inability to decide. The mind is filled with extreme doubt; you are so bewildered that you are paralyzed with fear.

There several derivative afflictions where these factors mix together. From anger, for instance, come wrath, vengeance, spite and envy, and from attachment such things as avarice, smugness, excitement and agitation.

Excitement is interesting, because from a Western point of view it is not abnormal or pathological. But it becomes so when you try to meditate...If you are too excited, too distracted by fantasy and so on, you simply cannot focus the mind.

The solution (to the problem of mental health) is seen in terms of the healthy, or wholesome, mental factors, which are the antidotes to the unhealthy ones. The first is clarity, or certitude. It is seeing things very clearly, a sharpness of mind that is antithetical to delusion.

The second is detachment, a non-grasping, non-clinging quality of mind. A detached attitude is one that lets go easily and does not cling.

A third wholesome factor is what might be translated as loving kindness. it is antithetical to hatred, to aversion. These three healthy factors oppose what are seen as the three roots of mental suffering: attachment, hatred and delusion.

There are other healthy wholesome factors: enthusiasm, or energy; faith or confidence--it is an intelligent, a questioning faith, not a blind faith--self respect; considerateness; conscientiousness; non-violence, or compassion, wishing everyone to be free from suffering; and equanimity.

This is an operational definition of mental health that says simply that the healthiest person is the person in whose mind none of the unhealthy, unwholesome factors ever arise. That is the ideal type, the prototype of mental health. The problem is, of course, that most of us, most of the time are in states where there is some mix of these things. So the question is, what to do?

Simply knowing a state is unhealthy does little or nothing to end it. If you resent your indecisiveness and wish it would go away, what you are doing is adding aversion and desire to the mix of mental states. So the strategy is a sort of an aikido approach, where you neither seek healthy states directly nor try to push them away. What you do is meditate." (11)

Desiring to experience these benefits, I was very interested in meditation in the 1970's and studied and practiced it intensely. When I earned a Bachelors Degree in Psychology in 1977, I focused my research on meditation. I learned to enter the profoundly blissful meditative state, but then did not keep up with it.

After practicing meditation for about ten years, I became bored with it and began to explore alternate ways to experience the meditative state. In the early 1980s I discovered the flotation tank. I had read Michael Hutchison's *Book of Floating*, and before long had my own float tank installed at my bodybuilding learning center, Zane Haven in Palm Springs. I must have floated over 1000 hours in the 2 years I kept the tank. The sensation of floating in 1000 pounds of epsom salt dissolved in 12 inches of 94 degree water was deeply profound and produced the meditative state in about 10 minutes. I usually would float an hour every day. I became very relaxed and the warm salt water released muscular tension stored in my shoulders, neck, and lower back.

The problem with the flotation tank was maintenance. Salt tracked all over the place and the salt water solution required constant attention. After two years I gave up and sold the tank. The deep relaxation I had achieved was continually being offset by the labor of working in a salt mine!

DICHOTIC AUDIO TAPES

During my floating sessions, I often listened to audio tapes and became interested in eliciting the meditative state with audio cassettes. Michael Hutchison had introduced me to the work of Dr. Lloyd Glauberman, a Manhattan clinical and sports psychologist, who had produced a series of audio tapes using multiple track stereo recordings which were designed to be listened to in the flotation tank. Glauberman called his method Hypno-Peripheral Processing or HPP. I was amazed at the deeply relaxing effects of listening to the tapes with headphones--they seemed to be able to trigger the meditative state automatically. Lloyd and I recorded several audio tapes together designed to facilitate deep relaxation and workout performance. Since then I've recorded several tapes with my wife Christine using a method similar to Glauberman's which I call Dichotics. Dichotic means listening to two messages at the same time, one in each ear through headphones.

Dichotic listening has been a valid method for studying the psychology of attention over the last three decades. Research has shown that people can be influenced by the meaning of words spoken in the ear they are not paying attention with even though they are unaware of the words. Our minds seem to extract meaning from such dichotic messages even though we may not remember hearing them (12,13,14).

While dichotic listening experiments are usually concerned with paying attention to one message at the expense of the other, Dichotics has no concern as to what the listener pays attention to. One may attend to the left ear message, the right ear message, both messages, or neither message--it simply doesn't matter. Dichotics is not used to study or train attention--quite the contrary. Dichotics makes use of the conscious mind's natural tendency to wander and not pay attention. Listening dichotically, a person eventually "lets go" of the effort of paying attention, relaxes, and becomes open to positive suggestion.

I'm often asked whether these tapes are "subliminal". Several studies show that subliminal messages recorded below the threshold of auditory awareness are not effective (15,16). Research has also revealed that people who believed they heard subliminal suggestions when they actually did not hear them were affected by this placebo effect and consequently resolved their problems (17).

There is nothing subliminal about dichotic audio tapes--you can hear everything. You simply cannot pay attention to all the information recorded on the multiple audio tracks, so you selectively attend to different parts of the tapes each time you listen. Suggestions conducive to relaxation, motivation, and performance become embedded in memory and pop into awareness when you're in a situation that calls for them (18).

I have found dichotic audio tapes useful both for relaxing after a workout as well as for producing a relaxed type of motivation when heard before a workout. It seems that even though one is able to follow the exact meaning of both of the stories from beginning to end, they do remember some of the words during workouts at key times, motivating them to stay mindful of their workout goals. Dichotic tapes divide the attention, trigger the meditative state, and optimize learning conditions while listening. Since focused attention is what's called for in a weight training workout--you must pay attention to what you are doing--dichotic audio tapes should be used before or after, never during a weight-training workout. Neither should they be listened to while driving an automobile or operating machinery.

Here is a sample script from a dichotic audio tape. The top line is heard in the left ear while the bottom line is heard in the right ear at the same time. The capitalized words which group together from each story form "embedded suggestions" which are heard as these words come together at points in time throughout the stories, such as "begin relaxation".

Now I'd like you to balance all the   RELAXATION
Just take your time....and as you   BEGIN   to feel

between the left side as well as the right side
you entire body becoming much more relaxed than ever

of your body. It's very important to   BALANCE
before on both left and right sides of   YOUR BODY

the relaxation that is expanding through   YOUR BODY
you know that cultivating this feeling......IS BEAUTIFUL

It's also a good idea to balance the total amount of
in many ways and the more you really practice relaxing

DEEP RELAXATION   you experience not only when you
THROUGHOUT THE DAY.... the easier and faster you will

are awake like   RIGHT NOW,   but also as you sleep
be able to   RELAX DEEPLY   whenever you want to in

because this is when   YOUR BODY   repairs itself.
a way that you always   WILL KEEP IMPROVING   quickly.

Your total relaxation must balance your total energy
In other words you need enough relaxation to balance

expended in exercise. And even though you may always
your energy output. This is due to the fact that

FEEL GOOD   during your workout, exercise is not really
WHILE YOU EXERCISE   you are in fact really tearing

relaxation which is the anabolic factor of bodybuilding
your body down. Exercise is catabolic and you need to

and it is this balance you keep between   EXERCISE
rest, relax, and recuperate to allow   YOUR BODY

and deep relaxation that we call homeostasis.
the opportunity to build and repair itself.

HIGH TECH MEDITATION

Realizing that mind/body mastery is the key to improved
mental concentration, increased energy, and peak performance
in workouts, my goal has been to master the mind/body
connection. My quest led me to discover that recent advances
in micro-electronics had given birth to compact computerized
training tools for mind/body exercises. These "mind/body
gymnasiums" are to mind/body exercises what sporting
equipment is to physical exercise. They work by using light

and sound. Training with these mind/body machines, I have quickly developed better meditative concentration and I'm realizing my goal of mastering the mind/body connection.

My method for mind/body mastery includes meditating with a mind/body machine and my dichotic audio tapes. The system I use is portable. I can carry this whole "gymnasium" in a belt wallet. For fitness enthusiasts as well as competitive bodybuilders, a winning training program exercises the mind together with the body.

Training for competition, I remember how difficult it was to keep a positive attitude. Doubts in the form of negative self talk, "mind movies" of gloom and doom, and worry about other competitors had a serious effect on my emotions unless I trained my mind as well as my body. In the late 1970's I didn't have the benefit of an electronic mind/body gym, so I disciplined myself to use meditation and the rudimentary audio tapes that existed at that time. Competing today, I would certainly take advantage of this electronic mind/body gym.

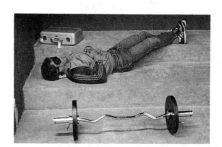
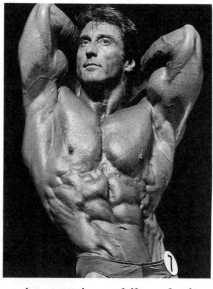

Frank visually mastering his posing routine while relaxing backstage before his last Mr. Olympia competition in 1983.

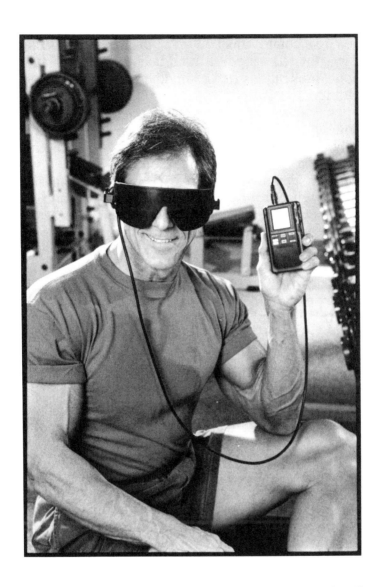

The compact **BRAINWARE 200** Mind/Body Exercise System is user friendly, completely programable, has built-in finger temperature sensor to gauge your mastery of your mind/body connection. Light screen & earphones built in a single headset produce an environment ideal for meditative concentration.

The light/sound meditation I practice uses scientific technology for developing mind/body harmony and has tremendous implications for the middle aged person practicing bodybuilding.

Anyone who exercises regularly realizes the importance of getting enough high quality sleep in order to recover completely and reverse the catabolic effects caused by training. In the past when I was training hard for competition, it was not uncommon to sleep nine or even ten hours each night in order to feel rested enough to experience peak performance in my workouts. Now, instead of spending more time in bed, I add thirty minutes a day of light/sound meditation in addition to my normal nocturnal sleep of six to seven hours. I feel that this time spent in meditation helps me elicit a state of relaxed alertness that carries over throughout my waking hours.

People tend to recycle unpleasant emotional reactions internally throughout the day. Meditation exercise is an effective way to interrupt the progression of negative emotions by saturating the senses with light and sound waves, which seem to help me wipe out negative self talk and undesirable mood loops.

RELAXED ALERTNESS

A recent study by Dr. Bruce Harrah-Conforth of Indiana University (19) suggests that light/sound machines may help an individual elicit simultaneous creative energy expenditure in conjunction with energy conservation. This is an ideal state of mind to practice visualization of your desired goals. I call this "relaxed alertness" which means just enough exertion for optimum performance in whatever task you are involved in-- alert, yet totally relaxed.

This state of relaxed alertness is the best way for the mature bodybuilder to train, for it is in agreement with the parsimony principle--no more exertion than is absolutely necessary. It also agrees with the Yerkes-Dodson Law which states that there is an inverted U-shaped relationship between exertion and task performance. Too little or too much exertion results in performance decrement, whereas just the right amount of exertion facilitates optimum performance. Furthermore, the more difficult and complex the task, such as in a weight-training workout, the lower the level of tension necessary for optimum performance (20). It's not necessary to bang your head against a wall to get psyched up for your training. Relaxed focused awareness always results in the best workouts.

Tension in muscles not used in a given task wastes energy (21). Such excessive tension may interfere with proper execution of movement in a weight-training exercise. Energy conservation techniques practiced prior to workouts can be beneficial in eliciting the right combination of relaxation plus exertion necessary for a great workout.

TRAINING WITH THE MIND/BODY GYMNASIUM

Using a body/mind gymnasium is actually a modern day form of meditation that combines age old visual and auditory meditative techniques. Visual meditative practices like gazing at colored discs called "kasinas", or into a flickering fireplace, or at a featureless plane or "ganzfeld" produce a calm yet heightened awareness. Auditory techniques such as chanting, repeating a positive affirmation or mantram, focusing on the sound of your own breathing, and contemplating the sound of ocean waves can be equated to the synchronized sounds of the mind/body gymnasium.

THREE STEPS IN MEDITATION

To achieve true meditation we must follow three steps:

1. Generate the meditative object to focus your concentration on, which can be an affirmation or your breathing.

2. Recycle this meditative object--repeat it over and over again to yourself for the entire length of the meditation which is usually 20 minutes or longer.

3. Pay attention to the meditative object--when your mind wanders, bring it back.

Being successful at meditation takes discipline and is best accomplished when you are practicing with a support group and a teacher. Practicing with people and a teacher can give you knowledge of results gained from meditation and help you improve your skill. This serves as positive reinforcement or a reward for your effort. It's difficult to continue doing something when you are unaware of your progress.

My own experience with meditation paralleled that of Charles Tart, a pioneer researcher in the psychology of consciousness:

"I had practiced various forms of meditation off and on for many years, but like most Westerners, had never been very successful at it. I sometimes half-jokingly (and sadly) described myself as an expert on the difficulties of meditation as a result of so much experience of my mind wandering off instead of focusing! In spite of my intellectual knowledge of the importance of meditation practice, some confusion as to just what to do and the consequent lack of results sapped my motivation, so I had not regularly practiced formal meditation for years until quite recently" (22).

I believe this lack of success many people experience with meditation is due to the lack of a proper tool. Just imagine trying to do bodybuilding without any barbells, dumb bells, benches, or exercise machines! For the same reason, meditation training with the electronic mind/body gymnasium is much easier. The three steps in meditation (generating, recycling, and paying attention to the meditation object) are achieved both internally as well as externally. You use an internal meditative object such as your own breathing, and you also take advantage of an external object: the synchronized pulsation of the light and sound from the electronic mind/body gym.

Meditating like this, I become centered and focused, with a sense of accomplishment from having achieved a higher state of consciousness. It is a very pleasant state to experience. Being an advanced meditator, I immediately know whenever I enter this state. Monks in the Himalayas have a unique way of demonstrating their achievement of the higher state of consciousness, and thus their mastery of the mind/body connection. These monks are able to show an increase in their fingertip temperature as a result of their mental power. To appreciate this ability, compare it with the last time you were about to shake hands with an important person and your hands became cold. The Himalayan monks illustrate how meditation training can help you take charge of your mind/body reaction. This is the power to be in control.

If you already meditate, begin your meditation with an electronic mind/body gym session. Program your unit to start at 18 to 20 hz, end between 7 and 10 hz, and continue meditating after the program ends. This is my post-workout meditation. You'll most likely experience a new level of higher consciousness, focused concentration, and increased alertness.

For my pre-workout meditation, I program my unit to start at 7, end at 18, and finally conclude at 13 hz. I also like to use the manual mode with 11 hz for visualization before my workout and 14 hz for pre-workout focus (23). Meditating with the electronic mind/body gym and my audiotapes before my workout, I visualize myself performing an ideal weight training session, getting a great pump on all my exercises. I also recollect what poundages and reps I did in my last workout on the bodyparts I'm training and see myself performing sets with perfect form using slightly heavier weights. Often ten minutes is all I need. After that I hit the gym and just do exactly what I've visualized.

The electronic mind/body gym is the main equipment in the small room adjacent to my weight-training gym. This small space is often called the "mind gym" (24), and is a favorite room for many people who come to Palm Springs to train with me. Here, we focus energy before workouts, as well as re-energize after hard training sessions. I believe all serious fitness facilities in the future will use this mind/body gym equipment.

My mind gym also contains a negative ionizer which can aid in improving memory and enhancing relaxation (25). The most effective one I have used is the *Elanra Therapeutic Ioniser* distributed by Bionic Products of America, Northfield, Illinois.

UNSTRESSING

I usually experience "unstressing" during a session of deep rest. This is a sudden release of stored tension in the form of involuntary twitches or body movement. The human mind is the repository of stress, tension, and mis-emotion, whether of physical or mental origin. During deep rest, the mind is liberated from stored tension through unstressing.

I also experienced a great deal of unstressing in using the flotation tank. I remember after lying in the salt water about one half hour, my shoulder or upper back would begin to twitch, and as I continued to relax, these involuntary movements would continue and intensify. Each movement seemed to be accompanied by a picture or impression of an incident in my recent past. Sometimes my whole body would convulse for several minutes. When I left the tank I felt extremely relaxed and much lighter.

My explanation for unstressing is that over a period of several weeks I built up a "body of negativity". By not fully paying attention and experiencing events and circumstances in my life, they got stored in my body. Soreness and tension seemed to build up very easily in the shoulders, neck, and lower back. I experienced pain here frequently when training hard and these were the areas that unstressed the most. Floating helped me dissipate this body of negativity and I became much more positive in my attitude. The phenomenon of unstressing helped me appreciate the need for experiencing deep rest on a regular basis.

Another device that seems to promote unstressing is the bio-circuit, a copper device that connects the lower back to the right hand and the lower neck to the left hand. The theory behind the bio-circuit is that it facilitates the flow of the body's own micro-potentials of electricity (26). Developed in the 1930's by L. E. Eeman, bio-circuits are based on the principle that when certain of the body's energy centers are linked together, the body's natural energy flow is enhanced. A recent study demonstrated that bio-circuit users developed slower EEG brain wave measures and lower EMG muscle tension measures during a normal 30 minute session on a copper bio-circuit (27).

SLEEP

While sleep itself is very important, unless you can fall asleep effectively, you won't experience optimum benefits. Audio tapes of environmental sounds like ocean waves or thunderstorms are especially soothing. One of the most powerful techniques for absorbing positive suggestions simultaneously while falling asleep during the evening or taking a nap during the day are Dichotic and Beat Frequency audio tapes. Since our brain wave activity slows down as we are falling asleep, it is reasonable to conclude that any technique that helps one slow down the mind's activity would also facilitate sleep.

Sleep is a period of restoration and repair during which anabolic physiological processes occur. Since sleep is constructive metabolism, there is an increased rate of cell division in adults. This effect is controlled by the secretion of growth hormone (GH) which increases the rate of cell division and promotes protein synthesis by facilitating the entry of amino acids into cells.

SLOW WAVE SLEEP & REM SLEEP

GH is secreted by the anterior pituitary shortly after the first occurrence of delta brain wave activity in slow wave or stage 4, the deepest level of sleep. Following slow wave sleep and GH secretion, brain waves frequencies increase to beta waves and a period of dreaming ensues. This is called REM (rapid eye movement) sleep, at which time protein synthesis within the brain increases. Studies suggest that REM sleep and the dreaming that occurs with it somehow assist people to deal with newly learned information that has emotional consequences. This may be why things seem less disturbing after a good night's sleep.

In the course of a normal night's sleep, GH begins to be secreted about one hour after the onset of sleep and lasts approximately one half or less. Then brain wave activity increases and a short period of dreaming occurs followed by another plunge into delta brain wave activity and the second phase of stage 4 sleep. This occurs about 90 minutes after its first appearance and GH is again secreted for about one half hour. This is followed by another ascent of brain wave frequency and a slightly longer period of dreaming. Dreams gradually grow longer as the night progresses, whereas no more stage 4 sleep and, consequently, no more GH release

210

occurs. So all of our GH release for one evening occurs within the first four hours when our sleep reaches its deepest levels.

Since the function of sleep is to repair the catabolic or destructive effects of activity during waking hours, it follows that sleep and exercise are related. Research indicates that slow wave sleep increased dramatically in athletes the two nights following an ultra-marathon (28). This shows that slow wave sleep is important for recuperation after strenuous exercise. In another study, it was found that people deprived of stage 4 sleep experienced muscle and joint pains and an overall increase in sensitivity to pain (29).

So even though more sleep is needed after hard workouts, what's really needed is more slow wave sleep. And it would seem that a person who trains hard will automatically spend more time in slow wave sleep to build and repair the body and offset the catabolic effects of vigorous exercise. With sleep being so important to a serious athlete, it is important not to let work or emotional issues keep us awake at night. I always clear my mind and focus my concentration on an inner sense of peacefulness in the evening before I go to bed.

PERSONAL GROWTH

Practicing both traditional as well as electronic meditation, and listening to dichotic and beat frequency audio tapes can provide benefits which lead to personal growth and power. As you become more proficient in your practice, not only will you become more calm and relaxed, but you will also develop more discipline in your workouts and in many other areas of your life. The experience of profound states of consciousness can lead to an awareness that there's something more to you than a physical body. This "something" is your Inner Self, the guiding, organizing factor of the psyche or total personality which motivates the journey toward full realization of what is possible during your lifetime. A great writer and teacher, Eknath Easwaran wrote:

"Most of us live on the surface level of consciousness, our grasshopper minds jumping from one subject to another, one desire to another, one distraction to another.   But as the mind is concentrated in meditation, we learn to extend our conscious control over successively deeper realms of consciousness, just as a diver learns to take deeper and deeper dives until he is able to walk about on the seabed.   In the climax of meditation, on the seabed of consciousness, we realize that we are not limited by the confines of the body or mind or even of the ego; we discover for ourselves the sources of abiding joy and infinite love that is our real nature." (30)

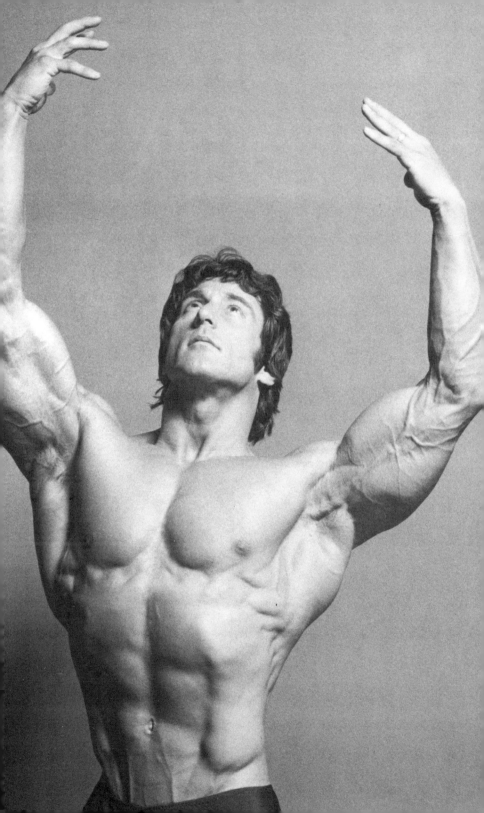

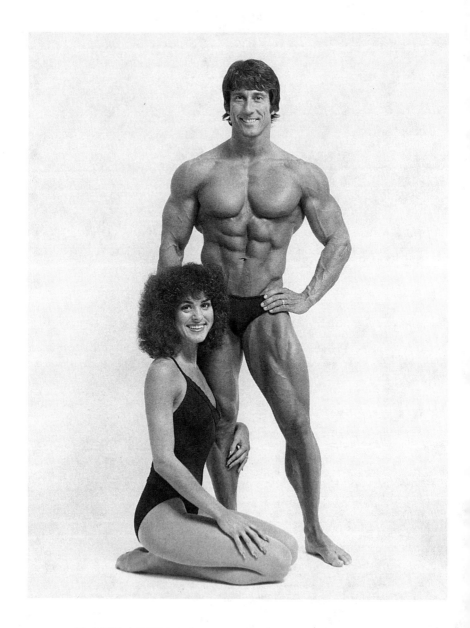

DAYS AFTER 1ST MR. OLYMPIA WIN, 1977

CHAPTER 11
BODYBUILDING, LOVE, AND SEXUALITY

"To be in love demands that the lover shall divine the wishes of the beloved long before they have come into the beloved's own consciousness. He knows her better than she knows herself; and loves her more than she loves herself; so that she becomes her perfect self without her own conscious effort. Her conscious effort, when the love is mutual is for him. Thus each delightfully works perfection in the other."

A. R. Orage

"Siempre fuiste la razon de mi existir
Adorarte para mi fue' religion . . ."

Carlos Almaran

"Love is, what you want it to be"

Alanah Miles

Does bodybuilding create better lovers? A lover is generally though of as a person who enjoys sex, the physical act of making love with another person. Although the spread of the HIV virus may have altered sexual behaviors, today's moral standards still condone sexual intercourse when two people love each other. So before we can know what constitutes a great lover as well as great love making, we must first understand what love is.

Love is one of the most important and powerful of all human emotions. The idea that there are many different kinds of love is not new. In ancient times, the Greeks described four different types of love: Eros or passionate, erotic love; Storge, or love between children and parents; Philia, meaning friendship or liking; Agape, a self-sacrificing, giving love.

EROTIC LOVE

Today when we speak of love, we usually refer to Eros, the beginning of which is characterized by a strong attraction to the physical appearance of the loved person (2). The culmination of the Eros instinct is the act of making love-- sexual intercourse using a variety of techniques. The erotic lover usually has an ideal partner in mind. In the case of the man, this is the anima, his archetype of perfect femininity which he projects to the woman he meets. The successful match of erotic lovers fulfills the condition that the female's ideal partner is her animus, or archetype of perfect masculinity the woman projects to the man. And usually, the better the body of the partner, the stronger the erotic attraction.

No doubt that a great body is a turn-on, one the opposite sex wants to touch and feel. Hormones circulate in the bloodstream and stimulate a sexual organ response. So developing a good body may be the first step toward building a more powerful sexuality. The right amount of exercise will also build endurance which improves sexual stamina resulting in the ability to prolong and enjoy climactic love making.

Prolonged love making is aerobic in nature, where heart rate hovers at target level, whereas intensely passionate love making becomes anaerobic, resulting in sexual climax--a peak physical experience. Indeed bodybuilding and sexual metaphors are often similar, such as "stay hard", "get pumped up", "push harder". In the book *Pumping Iron*, Arnold Schwarzenegger (3) describes the pump as being better than coming. The pump does provide a "body erection" by making the muscles bigger and harder. During a workout, physiological arousal occurs, muscles pump up and get harder, just as in the arousal of passionate love making, where full erection of both male and female sexual parts are maintained.

PASSIONATE LOVE IS A WORKOUT

According to some psychological theories (4,5) passionate love making occurs when two conditions exist simultaneously:

1. Partners experience intense physiological arousal, and
2. They apply a particular label -"love"-to the sensations they are experiencing.

This is a lot like a great workout where:

1. Intense heart pounding and sweating occur during a set, and
2. We label the pump we are experiencing as a "great workout".

So great sex and great bodybuilding workouts are both strong emotional experiences since each consists of a physiological state of arousal plus cognitive or mental labeling. This is why gyms are good places to fall in love. Men and women are in a state of physiological arousal from exercising and attribute these sensations, which they label as love (of the Eros variety), to attractive people with great bodies in the gym environment. This effect is called misattribution of arousal (6) and explains how gym romances get started and why coed gyms are so popular.

SEX, WORKOUTS, AND PARSIMONY

Sexuality and bodybuilding have parsimony in common. Bodybuilding can enhance sexuality and performance but only up to a point, which is the point just made: A well built body increases attraction to the opposite sex and has more stamina for sexual performance. So the right kind of training, nutrition, rest and recuperation, and attitude can make you sexier. But train too much, or don't eat enough nutritious foods and supplements, miss deep relaxation or don't get enough sleep,

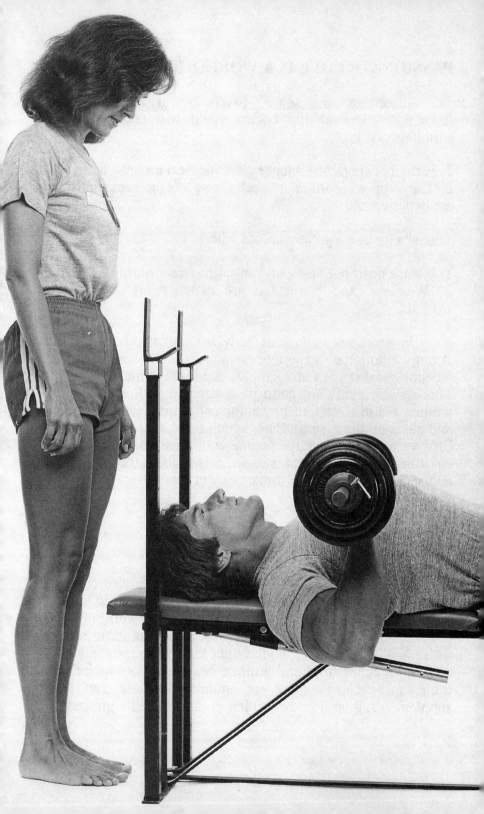

and entertain negative thoughts and watch your sexuality diminish. Balance is the key.

Sexual energy and workout energy all come from the same pool or reservoir. Over-train in your bodybuilding workouts and you'll have no energy left for sexual activity. Libido, life force, sexual drive, stamina, endurance are all names for the same quality. Sigmund Freud alluded to this idea that all energy is a derivative of sexual energy with his concept of "sublimation" where energy is displaced from a lower source, sexual or aggressive in nature, to a higher cultural expression. As part of this process, Freud saw sexual desire as a drive to discharge energy. (7)

Now whether bodybuilding is a sublimation of sexual energy is a moot question. The real issue is that both bodybuilding exercise and sexual activity are energy dependent. Use up this energy for either purpose and none remains for the other function. So take your choice.

I've known some real "studs", usually the guys who brag openly about sexual conquests, who do little of any kind of physical exercise except sex. They have no energy left for bodybuilding. None of their bodyparts are developed except one that was endowed by heredity. Bodybuilding, on the other hand, can develop all of your bodyparts except one. Bodybuilding may enhance sexual attraction but it does not improve sexual endowment.

Just as bodybuilding does nothing for the size of the male penis, it also does nothing for the fullness of the female breasts. Although breast measurement may increase with women who weight-train, this is due to the pectoral and back muscles increasing in size. The breasts are fatty tissue, and if too much weight is lost the breasts will reduce in size accordingly. I'm sure there would be more men and women practicing bodybuilding and less breast implants if this weren't true.

So balance your life by adjusting your priorities. Train and make love according to what is most important to you at the time. And don't expect to have all night love affairs if you are training for competition.

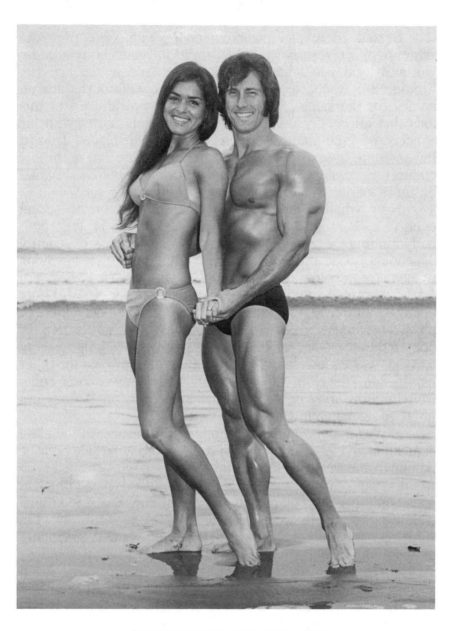

CHRISTINE & FRANK, 1970

B-LOVE, D-LOVE, MATURE & IMMATURE LOVE

Humanistic psychologist Abraham Maslow divides lovers into two categories: Being lovers (B-lovers) and Deficiency lovers (D-lovers). B-love is more independent, autonomous, individual, altruistic, generous, and fostering. Being lovers love with their entire being. D-love arises between two people because each seems to satisfy some needs the other has. Deficiency lovers love out of deficiency. B-lovers are selfless, D-lovers are selfish. (8)

A similar division is expressed by psychoanalyst Erich Fromm. He distinguishes between immature lovers who are highly dependent and live off each other, and mature lovers who show care, respect, responsibility, and knowledge of the loved person. Fromm describes sexual desire as a basic need to overcome isolation or a sense of separateness through erotic love and total union with the other. Loving is an art which is perfected through practice. (9)

Just as with continued practice, one can grow from an immature lover into a mature lover; one can become self-actualized in the passage from deficiency love to being love. I believe this passage from immaturity and deficiency to maturity and a higher level of being is analogous to the passage from bodybuilding as character armor to bodybuilding as character completion. It is part of the process of growing up by penetrating the muscular layer that supports the ego defenses which protect the immature person against suppressed feelings of fear, pain, inferiority, and shame. With maturity comes contact with the love contained in the heart of our being. The essence of love, which is the Inner Self is thus realized and the process of self actualization through sharing begins.

One morning I woke up and told Christine I dreamed we were walking through a city and found a lot of money in the form of $1000 bills. "I know" she said, "there were 21 of them. I was there too". We share the same dream is the metaphorical message. Dream life parallels waking life.

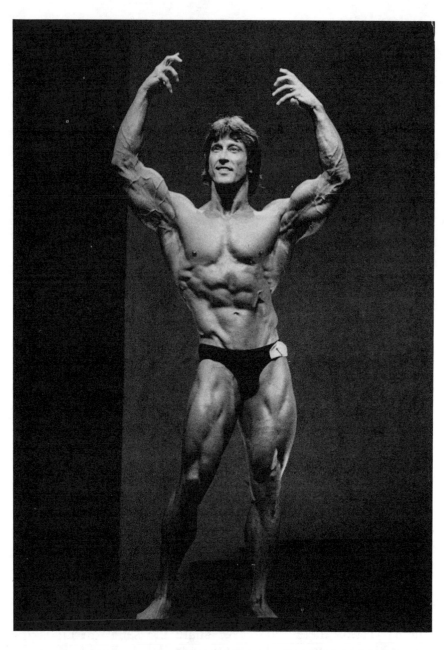

WINNING MR. OLYMPIA FIRST TIME, 1977

CHAPTER 12
ELEMENTS OF BODY TRANSFORMATION

"For the human body is not a finished, arrested form; it is ever in the process of becoming. That a healthy body kept in condition by care and exercise is more "body" than a neglected one is self-evident. But does the body reach its greatest dignity and perfection in the face and carriage of a man who lives among noble objects and pursues a thinking life, or in the trained and healthy but anti-intellectual and superficial man? If the question surprises us, it is because we are in the habit of looking at the human body much as we look at the animal body, as nature merely. But the human body is definitely determined by spirit. The face of a man who is passionately searching for truth is not only more "spiritual" than that of the man with a dulled mind, it is also more of a face, that is to say, it is more genuinely, more intensively "body". And there is not only more "spirituality" in the bearing of a man with a free and generous heart than in that of a crude and selfish person, there is a more responsive body. With man begins a wholly new scale of development. The body as such becomes more animated, more vibrating, as it is more strongly informed by the life of the heart, mind, and spirit."

Romano Guardini (1)

The body is transformed through disciplined wholistic practice. Bodybuilding in its fullest sense draws upon the human impulse toward wholeness which is evidenced as we grow in maturity. Perfecting the body through cultivation of our potential for physical, mental, emotional, and spiritual growth: This is **Transpersonal Bodybuilding**, a search for understanding of the whole of human psychological life.

What follows are my methods for getting the most out of your training by applying the finishing touches: dream-work, visual workout rehearsal, re-framing training motivation, my advanced exercise routine, the art of posing, bodybuilding as volitional suffering, and the dream body visualization. With consistent practice, these elements will radically transform the outward appearance of your body as well as your inner awareness. Taken in the order they are given, these elements of body transformation constitute a day in the life practice of bodybuilding as character completion.

DREAM-WORK

"Of the two dreams, night and day,
What lover, what dreamer, would choose
The one obscured by sleep?" (2)

Dreams give us messages about our emotional life that we may be unaware of during our waking hours. Many dreams are pictures of feelings. If we are not in touch with our feelings while awake, they often are expressed symbolically during REM sleep as dreams. Motifs for personal growth can be realized by paying attention to the content and feeling tone of a dream. Dreams help us heal by revealing a side of ourselves that we have been ignoring. In this sense, dreams are more real than waking life. They show us the true reality of ourselves by making us aware of our unowned parts. Do what you want with them, but dreams are the beginning in making us whole.

I mentioned the concept of the Inner Self in Chapter 1, describing it as the archetype of organization and personal growth. The following dream, which I call "The Butterfly in the Cave", put me in touch with my inner self and gave me important information about a transformative experience I was about to undergo at midlife:

As a boy I loved to hike in the mountains and
would often venture off by myself to explore nature.

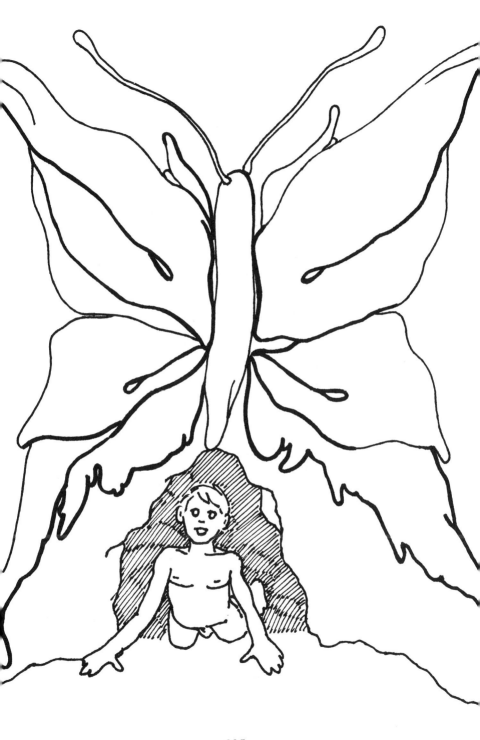

One day, I came upon the entrance to a cave that I had never seen before. At first, I was afraid to go inside because the opening was so small, but then curiosity got the best of me and I crawled into the small opening. It was dark, so I turned on my flashlight and saw that the passage led downward into the bowels of the earth.

After crawling on my hands and knees for some time, I entered a small room containing a cocoon. When I examined the cocoon, I saw that it was ruptured on the side. Then I heard a loud fluttering sound coming from above. I looked up and saw steps winding upward to a hole in the ceiling. Climbing the steps up through the hole in the ceiling, I entered a larger room and was amazed at the sight of a huge monarch butterfly with a 5 foot wingspan. I felt it was trying to scare me when it flew by and tapped me gently on the side of my head with its large wing.

I just stood in awe, witnessing the sight of the giant butterfly, wondering why a butterfly this big is in a cave deep inside the earth. I thought only moths hatched from cocoons inside caves. Still feeling the tap on the head, I noticed that there were several more compartments in the cave and the magnificent butterfly lived in one of them. The butterfly stayed very near to me for a while and then flew off into another compartment. I followed, but then the butterfly disappeared, so I followed a passage and eventually found my way out of the cave.

Exiting the cave, I noticed that this was not the same place I had entered. It looked very different, and as I began to look around, I discovered that I was on an island completely surrounded by water with no other land in sight. I gazed into the water and noticed that I was no longer a boy but had grown into a mature man.

After days of roaming the island, I eventually came to a building that seemed to be a school. There were many children inside sitting at desks, so I took a seat near the back of the classroom. I told a girl sitting next to me about the butterfly I had encountered in the cave, but the room was so noisy she didn't seem to hear me.

Then a curious thing happened. I had the feeling that I was dreaming and woke up within the dream! I was still dreaming but in a totally self aware way. Realizing that since this was my dream I could do whatever I wanted, I decided to take charge of the classroom. Moving to the head of the class, I called them to order and told them of my dream of the butterfly in the cave.

At this point I awoke and recorded the dream in my journal. This was a lucid dream which gave me a tremendous feeling of power and insight as I began to interpret the symbols. The cave symbolizes my unconscious mind. It was always there in the mountains not far from where I lived but I never realized it. The small opening was my opportunity to penetrate my character armor through self exploration. I used my flashlight to enlighten the darkness, that is, to make the unconscious conscious. The cocoon is symbolic of the ego and the material physical body and the change or metamorphosis it undergoes in the course of a lifetime. The caterpillar crawling on the earth incubates in a dark quiet place and grows into a totally transformed large beautiful creation who can fly. In life, the ego develops, changes, and emerges as a higher form of life, aesthetic with powers previously unattainable.

The impressively regal monarch butterfly is a symbol for the Inner Self. I made contact with it when its wing touched me on the head. It was a light tap on the side of the head that did something to my mind and belief system. Whereas I had formerly believed that inner exploration of the unconscious was opposed to physical exercise and led to stagnation, as expressed by the belief that cocoons hatching in caves turn into moths, just the opposite had occurred here. I had this dream in 1983 when I retired from bodybuilding competition. At this stage of my life it was necessary to get in touch with my Inner Self by exploring the depths of my unconscious mind. Since the physical body constitutes much of the unconscious, the message here was to look inside myself.

But after flying into another compartment in the cave, indicating that I must further explore my unconscious to stay near to my Inner Self, the butterfly was gone. Perhaps it had flown out of the cave. So I left the cave and came into the outer objective world in a different place and at a different time than when I went in. I went into the cave as a youth and came out as a mature person. I was on an island entirely surrounded by water symbolizing the limits of my personal world. The water was the collective unconscious, everything unknown to me in the universe, and I had no knowledge of what lay beyond it.

Back in everyday life, I looked around until I found a school. Taking a back seat, I became a student, but since the classroom was so noisy and out of control, I learned nothing, and couldn't share my dream with anyone. I finally had enough, awoke and realized the importance of communicating my dream to others. I moved to the head of the class, became a teacher, and told my dream to children of an impressionable age.

The dream doesn't end here, however. I've been telling people of all ages with active imaginations about getting in touch with their Inner Selves. Indeed, that's one of the goals for this book. Since dream life parallels waking life, waking up in my dream means that I am awakening in real life as well and living my dream.

With continuing dream work, self awareness increases and the language of dreams becomes less symbolic and more real. Puns, plays on words, multiple meanings, and metaphors are the language of the unconscious mind. As the unconscious becomes conscious, messages from the Inner Self are plainly stated. The skill is to remember these messages and pay attention to how you feel when you awaken. Dreams are as important as you allow them to be.

We have up to five dreams in one night, each increasing in length as the evening progresses. The final dream episode is about one hour long and is the one I pay the most attention to. A balance must be maintained between dream life and waking life so as not to be overwhelmed by unconscious contents, so don't be in a hurry to understand everything. To get started in dream-work, I suggest you read a good book about the subject. My favorites are *Lucid Dreaming* and *Exploring the World of Lucid Dreaming* by Stephen LaBerge.

If you don't remember your dreams upon awakening, just ask yourself how you feel and write this feeling along with anything you can remember in your dream journal. Christine and I often tell our dreams to each other and have found this to be an effective way to feel better in the morning. Writing or talking about dreams releases pent up feelings and we seem to function better during the day. On the other hand, If we don't record or discuss our dreams and let them slip from awareness (especially if our dream is unpleasant), we often experience the same emotional mood of the dream during the day and feel out of sorts or depressed. If your dream seems incomplete, you can finish it any way you would like. After all, the dream is your creation.

Psychologists believe that emotions are cognitively mediated. We feel a body sensation and then we label it with our thoughts. This is exactly what we do when we interpret our dreams. We give meaning to the sensations, sights, and sounds we experience in our dreams. Be optimistic in dream interpretation: by changing your mind you can change your mood.

VISUAL REHEARSAL

In a sense, visual rehearsal is like dreaming about activities you are planning by seeing yourself performing exactly as you would like to. It is a great way to improve your mood and feel good about your workout before you do it. I often find myself doing this automatically without any conscious effort. It is a way to get psyched up for your workout. To practice it more formally, sit in a comfortable position, close your eyes, and see yourself entering the gym and doing your first exercise and corresponding stretch immediately afterward. Go through all your exercises in this fashion and decide what weights you will use and how many reps you will do on each set. Is there any bodypart that needs extra work? See yourself doing extra sets or adding another exercise for this area.

It's not necessary to go through every set of each exercise in your pre-workout visual rehearsal. When I did this I seemed to lose some enthusiasm for my workout. The idea is to hold a tentative picture in your mind before you begin training, and then let your workout unfold according to your instincts when you are in the gym.

After my workout, I recollect each exercise, set, number of reps, weights used and write them in my workout journal or diary. Since I have been doing these exercises so long I remember everything. By doing this, I re-experience my workout and reinforce the association between the proper performance of the movement with the pump I achieved in the session. This also connects with the sensation I am experiencing in the muscle as I write up the workout. After I finish, I get a feeling of satisfaction, not to mention a record that I can refer back to in the future for feedback and motivation.

RE-FRAMING TRAINING MOTIVATION

The desire to become a champion bodybuilder can emerge at any stage of life. How you train depends upon when this occurs, since you have more energy when you are younger. Bodybuilding is a means to strengthen your ego. The task of youth is to develop and fortify one's developing ego by participating and winning competitions. During my youth, I did this through the struggle of bodybuilding contests, finally winning the Mr. Olympia at age 35 after twenty one years of training.

The lesson I learned from competition was not to give up. I certainly lost more contests than I won and it seemed that these losses gave me motivation to do better the next time around. I was able to change my perspective by making the loss mean: "I have another chance at winning, so I will get a new training plan to improve my weakpoints, and come back and win." This practice of extracting the energy tied in losses and turning it into positive motivation is called re-framing. The basic re-framing question I asked myself after a defeat was "How can I use this experience in a positive way to help me grow?"

Sometimes it was hard to answer this question right away and I found myself blaming the judges or circumstances I thought were beyond my control. After being negative for a while, I saw the folly of it all and was able to laugh at my negative attitude and behavior. Seeing the humor in a negative situation is often the first step in re-framing. After a good laugh I was able to calm down and calculate an intelligent strategy for winning. Opportunity always presented itself again. My mother used to tell me: "God closes one door and opens another."

Re-framing losses in this manner worked very well for my entire competitive career, the challenge of competition motivating me to prove myself again and again. But the task I faced when I retired from active competition was how to motivate myself to keep training and improving. After long reflection, I began to realize that the only real competition was with myself, my previous bests. Competition with others forced me to train harder--I came out of myself to meet this challenge. This is external or extrinsic motivation which relies on deficiency. I train harder so that I can improve what is lacking in my body so I will compare favorably to others. Maslow would call this D-motivation, or motivation out of a sense of need or deficiency.

Now, at midlife, my goal is not competition with others, but with myself. Whereas competition with others did force me to train harder during my contest training season, competition with myself motivates me to balance my training efforts over the entire training year by relying on my seasonal approach (see Chapter 8). I realized that comparison with others is based on value judgement. It is easier and more objective to compare changes in yourself as evidenced in photos than it is to compare yourself to other bodies. Comparing your best physique to another person's is like comparing apples to oranges. It's a matter of taste, preference, opinion.

Inspiration comes from role models whose lives serve as examples for others. Sri Chinmoy, a spiritual teacher who also practices bodybuilding is such a person whose words and deeds have uplifted many athletes:

> "Each new day beckons you to walk on the road of self-transcendence. When we transcend ourselves, we do not compete with others. We compete only with our previous achievements. And each time we surpass our achievements, we get joy...Life is nothing but a perpetual possibility."(3)

At this stage in my life most of my ongoing training is intrinsically motivated by competition with exceeding my previous bests. An important point I came to realize was that my previous bests weren't always found in my physical body. I've found there is always some aspect of my workout, nutrition, relaxation, and attitude that I can improve. Now instead of being motivated by deficiency I am motivated by my successes. The transformation process which occurs at midlife involves successfully changing your motivational system from external to internal. It's not always easy, but it is possible by applying the techniques elaborated in this chapter. Your best can always get better!

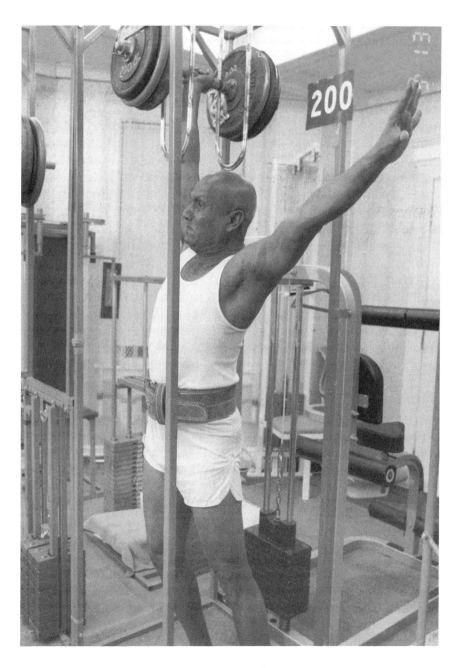

SRI CHINMOY

THE ADVANCED ROUTINE

Whether you are a youth motivated by competition or an intrinsically motivated bodybuilder at midlife, the advanced routine which follows is designed to get you into shape more quickly than any of the programs previously given. Don't just jump into it without progressing through the 3 way split routine of Chapter 6. This would result in excessive soreness and increase the possibility of over-training and injury.

My advanced bodybuilding routine is an extension of the 3 way split routine given in Chapter 6. The main difference is the advanced routine contains more exercises and lots of super-sets. A super-set is two exercises done one right after the other without resting. Super-sets save time by intensifying the workout and build muscular definition. The program also contains tri-sets, that is, three exercises in a row done without resting until all are completed. It takes a lot of stamina to tri-set successfully, but the results are quick and dramatic. Super-sets and tri-sets limit the amount of weight you are able to use on the exercises which follow the first exercise. This kind of training works well when practiced with the Time Star method described in Chapter 7.

This program is practiced on a four day cycle, training three days in a row and resting the fourth day. You can train once a day, or you can come back to the gym for a second session where you work abdominals and do aerobics. This routine is designed to bring the body to absolute peak condition and should not be practiced for more than 8 to 12 weeks. Doing it any longer may result in over-training. It's a good idea to take an extra day off if you are feeling really sore and tired. Since many of the exercises are done on machines, you will need a well equipped home gym or health studio to perform this routine. The deep relaxation techniques described in Chapter 10 are essential to help conserve energy necessary for hard training sessions. I do 3 sets of each exercise, eventually progressing to 4 sets on some of the exercises as my energy and enthusiasm permit. Here's my program: (I will illustrate only the new exercises denoted by *.)

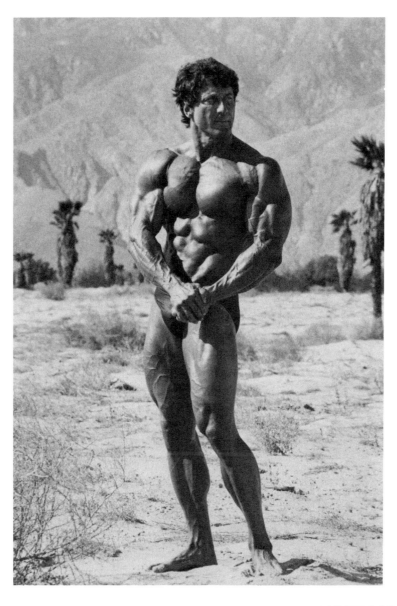

TWO WEEKS BEFORE 1982 OLYMPIA, WEIGHT 205

See Chapter 6 for description of the other movements and Chapter 3 for the stretches.

DAY 1 - BACK, BICEPS, FOREARMS

Back

Front pulldown super-setted with
Cable crossover behind neck * & 2 arm lat stretch

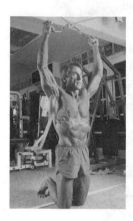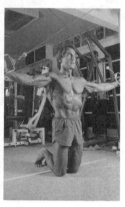

Seated low cable row super-setted with
Bent over rear cable raise* & 2 arm lat stretch

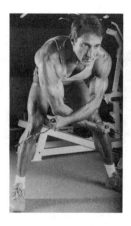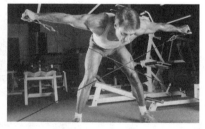

1 arm DB row super-setted with
1 arm cable row* & 1 arm lat stretch

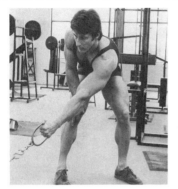 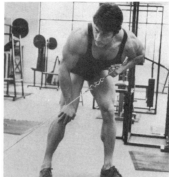

Biceps

Bistar curl * (with the rubber pad behind wrist, curl upward)

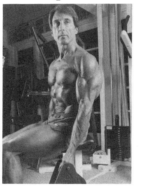

super setted with: DB concentration curl *

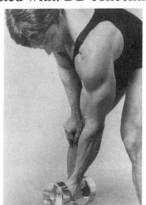 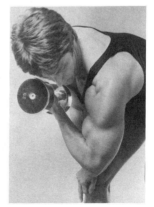

Face down incline DB curl super-setted with:
Preacher cable curl* & pronated arms back stretch

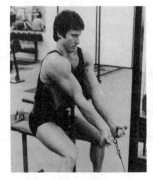 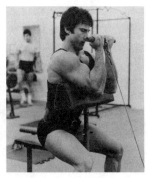

Forearms

Reverse wrist curl * tri-setted with

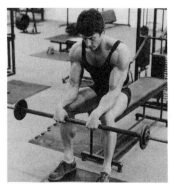 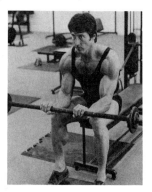

Barbell wrist curl, and
Hand gripper * & pronated arms back stretch

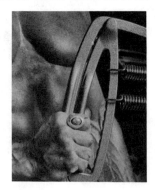

DAY 2 - CALVES, THIGHS

Calves

Standing calf raise tri-setted with
Seated calf raise and
Incline calf raise with *Soloflex Rockit* * & calf stretch

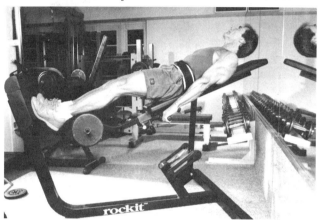

Thighs: all exercises are super-setted

Standing one leg curl *

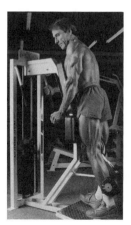
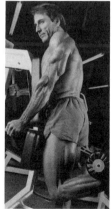

super setted with Hip Machine * (for outer thigh)
& 1 leg up stretch

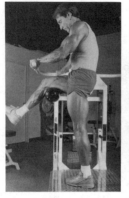 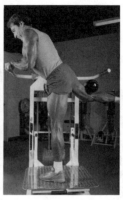

Leg extension & 1 leg back stretch
super setted with Leg curl & 1 leg up stretch

Leg Blaster squat
super setted with Stairclimber (fast for one minute)

DAY 3 - CHEST, SHOULDERS, TRICEPS

Chest/front deltoids: (all exercises are super-setted)

30 degree incline DB press super-setted with
Cable crossover* & doorway stretch

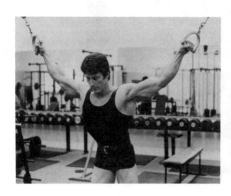 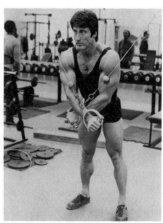

Pec deck * super-setted with

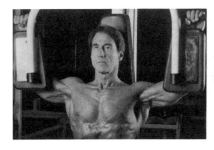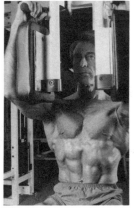

Front press machine* and doorway stretch

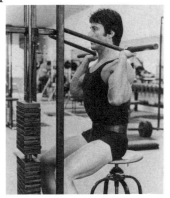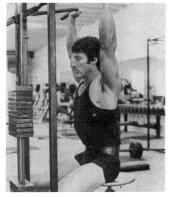

Dip machine* super-setted with

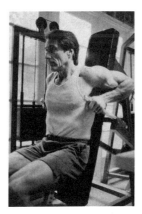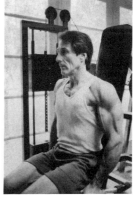

Rear delt machine* & doorway stretch

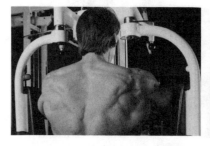 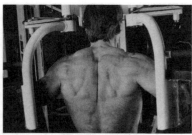

DB pullover super-setted with
Stiff arm pulldown *

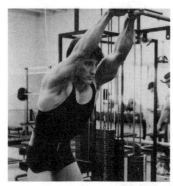 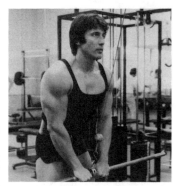

Shoulders/triceps: (all exercises are super-setted)

1 arm DB tricep extension super-setted with
Bistar 1 arm side raise * & 1 arm shoulder stretch

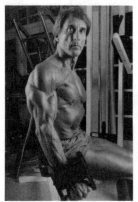 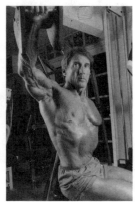

Triceps pressdown super-setted with
Pronated DB side raise * & rear delt stretch

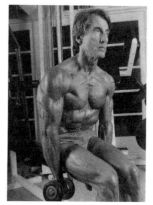 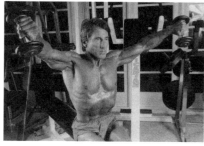

1 arm triceps cable kickback * super-setted with

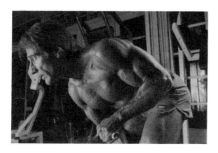 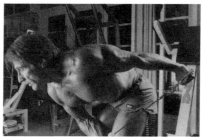

1 arm side cable raise * & arms back stretch

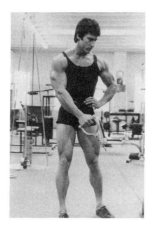 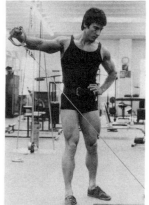

ABDOMINALS AND AEROBICS

I like to do the weight training part of this workout in the morning and come back to the gym for one hour in the afternoon for ab work and aerobics. I gradually keep adding reps, sets, and new exercises until I'm doing 1000 reps daily on abdominals. This is a lot of ab work but the results are fantastic! It takes me about 40 minutes non-stop to complete the ab routine:

Pulley knee in * - 4 sets of 25 to 50 reps *

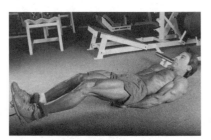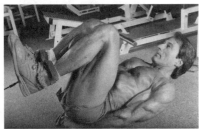

Crunches - 4 sets 25 to 50 reps super-setted with
Hanging knee up * - 4 sets 25 to 50 reps

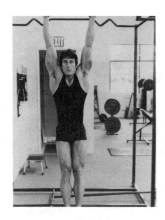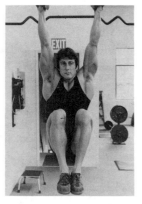

Incline leg raise - 4 sets 25 to 50 reps super-setted with
Two Arm cable crunch * - 4 sets 25 to 50 reps *

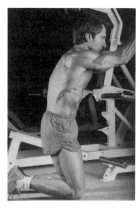 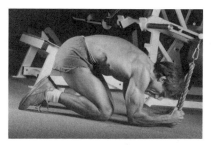

Seated twist - 4 sets 50 reps supersetted with
1 arm cable crunch * - 4 sets 25 reps each side *

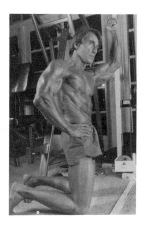 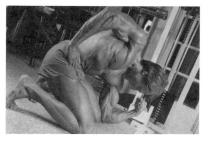

Hyperextension - 2 sets of 25 reps

Day 1 Aerobics - 10 to 20 minutes of rowing
Day 2 Aerobics - 20 to 30 minutes of treadmill
Day 3 Aerobics - 15 to 20 minutes of Stationary Bike

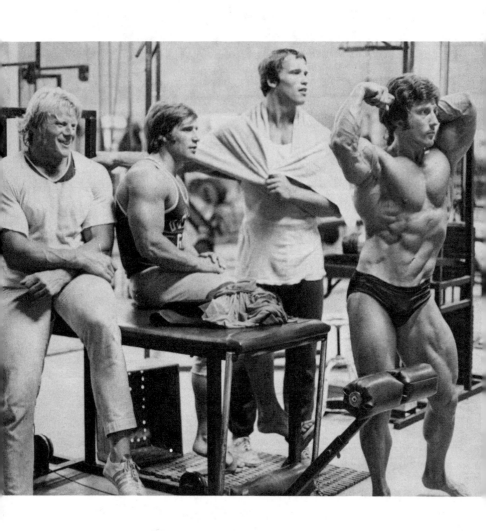

DAVE DRAPER, SERGE JACOBS, AND ARNOLD CHECK
OUT FRANK'S POSING AT GOLD'S GYM, 1970

THE ART OF POSING

Bodybuilders are the only athletes who prepare for competition one way but compete in a completely different way. To build a great physique it is necessary to train scientifically with weights, practice stretching, aerobics, good nutrition, and deep relaxation. But to win a physique contest the bodybuilder must master the art of posing.

Posing is like moving sculpture. The statue is alive and assumes artistic positions while tensing all the muscles of the body simultaneously, except the facial muscles. The movement from pose to pose is dynamic yet graceful and the well developed physique is displayed to advantage.

There are two basic styles of physical development in bodybuilding as exemplified by the classic sculptures, "The Farnese Hercules" and Michaelangelo's "David". Arnold Schwarzenegger is the best example of the first, whereas I am of the second category. Since the history of bodybuilding has been dominated by the massive herculean body and still is, many think that the physique must be massive to be impressive. Bodybuilding would probably be even more widely accepted if more of its advocates trained to develop more muscular detail, definition, and better proportion. This always was my strategy for winning since I was never a physical giant.

The practice of posing is the way to develop such muscular detail. By tensing the muscles and holding the pose for progressively longer periods of time, the bodybuilder develops great control over his body. Eventually, one can tense all the muscles yet be completely relaxed. This is the paradox of being in ultimate muscular condition and is related to the concept of relaxed arousal described in Chapter 10. This ultra-fine condition results from the isometric effect of holding each pose.

Isometric contraction is exercise without movement. Posing is both static and kinetic, tension plus movement, sculpture dancing. The finished look resulting from continued practice of posing bodybuilders call "muscle maturity".

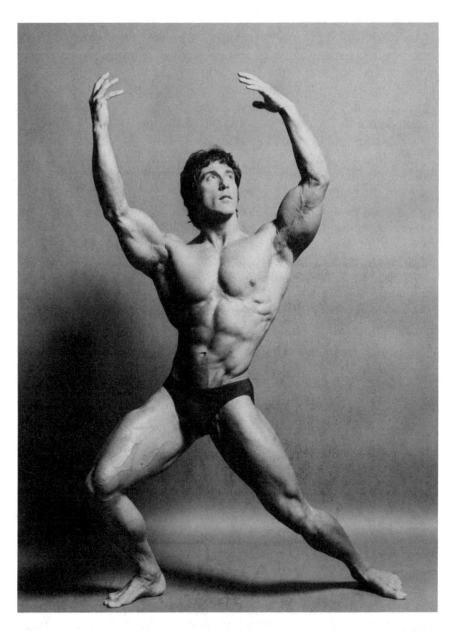

FRANK IN 1976

It's the look that wins competitions. But even if you are not interested in competing in bodybuilding events, the practice of posing can be a useful way to measure the results of your training. All you need is a bathing suit and a camera.

Measuring progress is an important part of bodybuilding which provides such knowledge of the results of your training. There are many ways to measure progress which involve the use of numbers: You can use a tape measure to see how many inches you've lost around your waist or gained in your arms; you can weigh yourself; you can calculate your percentage of bodyfat with calipers or by the water displacement method. But with these methods all you get is a number--a description of reality, not reality itself. If these numbers were so important they would be part of the judging criteria for bodybuilding competition. In such competitions, judgement is based solely on appearance.

Everybody who trains is interested not only in feeling better but also in looking better. The best way to measure how you look is with photographs, specifically color slides because you can project them to life size. Looking in the mirror is not an accurate assessment of your appearance because you see what you expect to see. Your appearance is distorted by the bubble of perception called your self-image. We cannot see ourselves accurately. An egoist always sees something better than what's really there, an anoretic, no matter how emaciated, always sees a fat person.

I would go so far as to say that no one possesses full body awareness. It's just not possible since judgement of ourself is always subjective. Furthermore, there are parts of our bodies we never see, such as our back. Viewing color slides of ourself taken at one month intervals throughout our training year will give us an accurate idea of what we really look like, providing photographic conditions are held constant. Before you can change something you must first become aware of it. Slides give feedback on what bodyparts are progressing and what parts are stuck. With this awareness you can modify your training accordingly.

A technique I used involving color slides in preparing for the Mr. Olympia competition was to project recent color slides of my physique onto a large sheet of paper and draw my current form on the paper. Over the next two weeks I continued to erase pre-existing lines and add new ones. My goal was to coincide the changing real images on film with the images drawn from my imagination. By making this connection between my active imagination and current physical self as portrayed on film, I changed quite rapidly over a period of 12 weeks. The artwork became a blueprint for my future physical development. Imagination is indeed the will of things.

THE COMPULSORY POSES

Taking photos means you must learn a few simple poses in addition to standing normally from the front, back, and sides. The basic poses are:

Front double biceps pose   Front lat spread

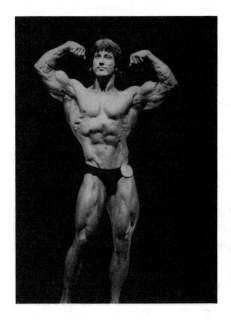
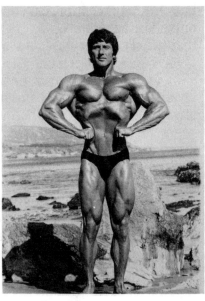

Side chest pose

Back double biceps

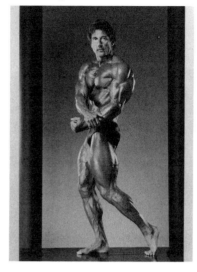
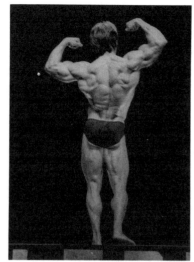

Back lat spread

Side triceps pose

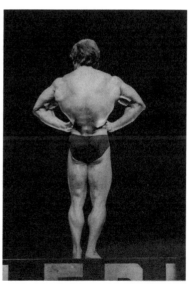
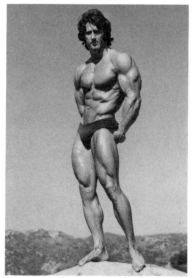

Abdominal pose

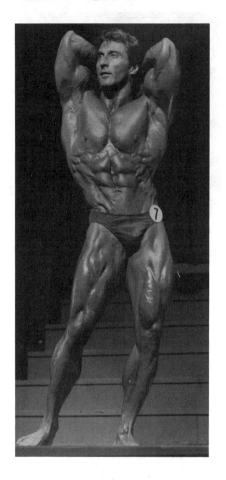

Standing relaxed

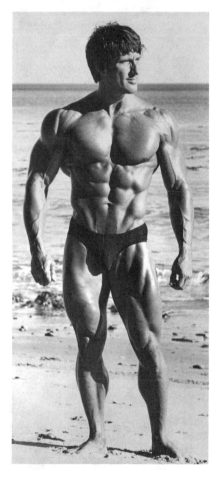

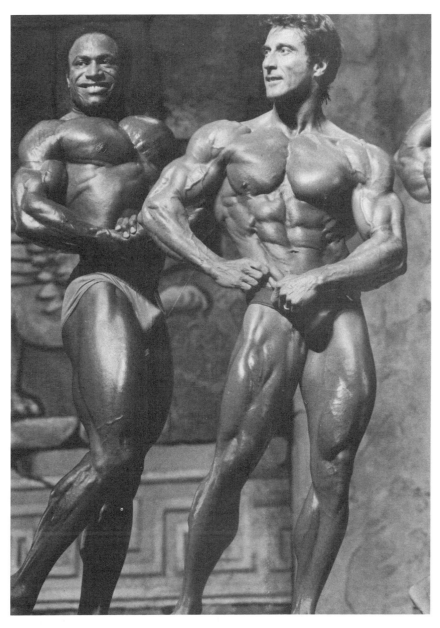

POSEDOWN AT 1983 MR. OLYMPIA. THIS WAS
FRANK'S LAST COMPETITION AT AGE 41 & LEE
HANEY'S FIRST APPEARANCE IN THE OLYMPIA.

Posing is what competitive bodybuilding is all about, but even if you aren't interested in competition, I know you want to assess your progress, and photos of your poses are the best way to measure it. You'll also get a great isometric workout from holding the poses and this will help improve muscular definition.

FREE POSING

The other kind of posing that is necessary to learn if one wants to compete in bodybuilding contests is called optional or free posing. Every free pose is a modified version of a previously described compulsory pose. Looking at the pictures in bodybuilding magazines can give you an idea of how many poses are possible. Each pose expresses an attitude-- "posing language"; the side chest pose, pride; front lat spread, overpowering self-confidence; front double biceps, completeness; most muscular pose, hardness, durability; arms overhead, victory. In effect, the champion's posing routine reflects a full range of emotional expression.

Bodybuilding competitions were always sculpture contests for me. The photographs of the contests have very strong survival value as they become permanent records of the events which are recorded by the bodybuilding media. These photos provide the images for aspiring bodybuilders to visualize. As they are continually exposed to them, their impact registers an indelible impression on the unconscious minds of aspiring bodybuilders and influences their behavior.

Photos of yourself will enable you to look at your body objectively. Looking outside yourself, you see the image of your body as something external to yourself. As you continue to take photos every few weeks, you will see your body change externally on the photos. This in turn changes your body image. You can use these improving photos of yourself as concrete images for the bridge you build in the Dream Body Visualization coming up in this chapter.

Some tips on taking good color slides are: always use the same film (I like Fuji Velvia), and the same 35mm camera with the same lens (a normal lens is fine. I like a 85 mm lens also. Never use a wide angle lens). Pick an undistracted background and have your photographer shoot your body full frame with vertical format. Take the photos with the sun at about a 45 degree angle with the horizon. Avoid mid-day directly overhead sun as it creates dark shadows. Mornings or late afternoons are best. Decide on the time and then always take the photos at this time, allowing for seasonal variation in the position of the sun, for the best comparisons. If you decide to use color photos instead of color slides, you can paste the photos into your workout diary at the times they were taken. Over time, you'll be able to compare how you look with what you do in your training.

Bodybuilding is about images. More attention should be given to using visualization regularly to bring these images to life. Since action always seems to follow thought, what you see is what you get!

VOLITIONAL SUFFERING

"The circumstances which a man encounters with suffering are the result of his own mental inharmony..Suffering is always the effect of wrong thought in some direction. It is an indication that the individual is out of harmony with himself, with the Law of his being. The sole and supreme use of suffering is to purify, to burn out all that is useless and impure. Suffering ceases for him who is pure. There could be not object in burning gold after the dross had been removed, and a perfectly pure and enlightened being could not suffer." (4)

In essence, the mature bodybuilder becomes a craftsman whose central task is the creation of himself through practice, rest, repetition and patience. This patience is reflected in the process of volitional suffering as it operates in a bodybuilder's training. We have a choice as we age: don't exercise and suffer

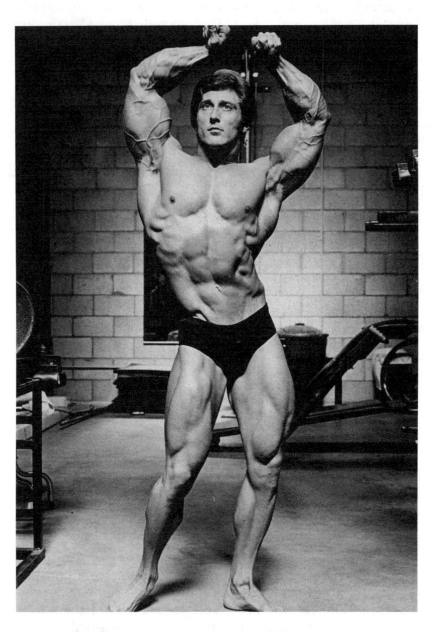

AGE 28, AFTER WORKOUT AT GOLD'S GYM, 1969

the physical liabilities of aging against your will, or exercise and consciously choose how you suffer. Conscious suffering, which is the result of choosing how you train, always results in growth.

We spoke of bodybuilding exercise as destructive metabolism, the process by which the body is systematically micro-traumatized by vigorous exercise. Destruction is the first step in the process of creation. Catabolic effects like capillary damage and waste product build-up caused by the stress of weight training are counteracted with the anabolic agents of good nutrition and deep relaxation. Consequently, the body adapts by becoming more fit.

The theme of suffering is succinctly expressed in the bodybuilding metaphor, "NO PAIN, NO GAIN". Without suffering, no growth is possible. Flesh must be broken down in order to be reformed into something new. This can also be a potentially dangerous metaphor because people have different ideas of what constitutes pain. For me, pain has a negative connotation indicating injury. I prefer the expression, "NO PUMP, NO GAIN".

I also prefer the word "stimulation" to pain. It's a good idea to understand the stimulation that occurs during a set of an exercise. As you continue to do reps in good form, the first sensation you should feel is a pump, providing you are concentrating deeply on the movement and doing it correctly. The inflated feeling of the pump should occur on your last few reps and become even more apparent as you rest and stretch between sets. If you were to keep doing reps, either by reducing the weight or having someone assist you raise the weight, you feel a "burn" which is caused by waste product build-up (mainly lactic acid) in the muscles. As you rest and stretch, this burn turns into a pump and the muscle feels expanded and bigger since it is swollen with blood.

At some point along the way between pump and burn is positive failure-- you cannot complete the positive phase of the repetition, that is, you can't get it up. Even more severe than positive failure is negative failure or using so much weight that you fail on the negative phase of the rep and you can't get it down. Although negative failure builds muscle size and strength even more than positive failure, it is very dangerous and should be avoided if you want insurance for training longevity. This kind of training and the heavy weights used to induce it really taxes the joints and ligaments.

Suffering is also reflected in bodybuilding's many aggressive war metaphors: bombing, blitzing, and blasting the muscles refers to hard training; cannonball deltoids are the epitome of shoulder development; bodybuilders refer to arms as guns (the title of Larry Scott's book on arm training is *Loaded Guns*): the race to bare arms explains why biceps and triceps are such popular bodyparts and symbols of strength. When going to war you bear arms--anatomically, you bare your arms for combat. Such war metaphors are misleading since war implies killing or at least injury. This is definitely in violation of the parsimony principle which says make the most gains from the least amount of training-- intelligent training, not the over-training inspired by such aggressive figures of speech. You don't have to kill yourself to make progress.

Successful bodybuilding is about re-framing suffering, that is, developing a new perspective about the effects of hard training. Since we can't avoid suffering in life, all we can do is change our attitude toward it. Just how the stress of a workout effects us is mediated by our perception and appraisal of how we feel afterwards. The successful bodybuilder is one who is happy as a result of being sore the day following a workout. This intentionally created soreness or volitional suffering, means knowing just how much training is enough. Too much soreness means over-training or injury, too little means no progress.

So have the right attitude toward soreness, because without it growth is impossible. Much of the time in our moments of ordinary awareness our body whispers its wishes to us which often go unheeded. Soreness is your body shouting to you, "I had a great workout!" You can't help but hear it. This dichotic tape script when listened to with headphones can help reframe your attitude toward soreness:

DICHOTIC REFRAMING SCRIPT: The top line is heard in the left ear and the bottom line is heard in the right ear simultaneously:

As the man got ready for his workout, he knew that
Even though the young woman had never flown a

he had to train hard enough to get **SORE** from
glider before, she was thrilled to **SOAR** among

his training in order to make progress. So he
the clouds with her dog as a companion. Being

concentrated on every rep, making sure that his
up in the air like this, riding the updrafts and

negatives were always slower that his positives.
downdrafts of wind that would come her way

He knew he'd get **SORE** if he trained this way.
enabled her to **SOAR** along the mountainside.

And from that moment on, he was sure that he
What is this wonderful sensation I'm feeling right

would always train hard enough for **SORENESS**.
now she said to herself, might it be **SOARNESS**?

Learning to modulate soreness is what making gains is all about.   Modulation means to regulate by changing the frequency and intensity. You regulate the catabolic effects of your workouts by training more or less frequently.   You control exercise intensity by training with less rest between sets, using heavier weights, and doing more sets and reps, that is you do more work in less time. When this is properly done in training, suffering becomes stimulation, and with it comes the power and fun of creating your own living sculpture: YOU!

Since basal metabolism slows with age, a major goal for ongoing training is to slow down body attrition. As you get older there is a tendency to lose lean body mass. This muscle mass is important to keep one's resting metabolic rate elevated. For every pound of muscle lost with age, we burn about 50 fewer calories per day. With muscular atrophy comes fat hypertrophy. By age 90 the average non-exercising person has one third of the muscle mass he or she had at age 20! So as you get older, even staying the same means making progress. But this doesn't mean that you should be content to stay the same in your training.

There is an order of bodybuilding progress: to improve is best, to maintain is OK, and to regress is undesirable. Some regression, however, is inevitable from day to day. Have a great workout, set a personal record, but don't expect all you subsequent training sessions to be as good. What happens in such situations is called "regression toward the mean". Great days are followed by mediocre days-- it all averages out. It's what you do most of the time that counts in the long run. By using my seasonal approach to training intensity described in Chapter 8, you can set and reach short term goals and meet your long term yearly goals according to plan.

THE DREAM BODY VISUALIZATION

"According to Homer, man has a dualistic existence, the one in his visible appearance, the other in his invisible image which becomes free only after death--this, and no other is his soul. In animate man there dwells as a strange guest, a more feeble Double-- his other self in the form of his Psyche-- whose kingdom is the world of dreams. When the conscious self sleeps, the Double works and watches." (5)

Your dream body **is** your Double. This dream body is the image you see as yourself in your dreams. With dream-work you can change your dream body and consequently change your physical body. Here is the fundamental visualization technique for doing this:

About 20 or 30 minutes before bedtime, sit in a comfortable chair or lie down in bed, close your eyes, and focus your inward vision on your forehead. Imagine your forehead as a large movie screen. See your body as it is right now, filling the entire movie screen. Just take your time...and see yourself as you look right now. Look at all the parts of your body: your face, head, neck, shoulders, chest, back, arms, elbows, forearms, wrists, hands...your stomach, hips, buttocks, genitals, thighs, knees, calves, ankles, feet, and toes...that's right...Now as you continue to hold this image of your body as it is right now in your awareness, move it to the left side of your large movie screen. Keep looking up and to your left, continuing to imagine your body as it is right now, seeing everything about your body that you are not satisfied with and want to change. Consider every detail of each bodypart..................good.

Now look up and to your right visual field and imagine the future of your body, the body of your dreams. It may be someone else's body that you admire, your role model or bodybuilding idol, and imagine what it feels like to have this body-- the strength, the exhilaration, full of energy yet deeply relaxed. And from your position in your ideal dream body in your upper right visual field, look to your left and invite your old body to join you. Together, your dream body and your former body begin constructing a bridge, a bridge from the past to your future. The work of constructing this bridge involves all the exercises, foods, supplements, thoughts, words, actions, sleep, dreams, and meditations that you can possibly do to build your perfect body. This work is made easier because both your former body as well as your dream body are working together, doing exactly what is necessary in the right amounts to transform you. And as your bodies continue to work together building the bridge to transformation, they move

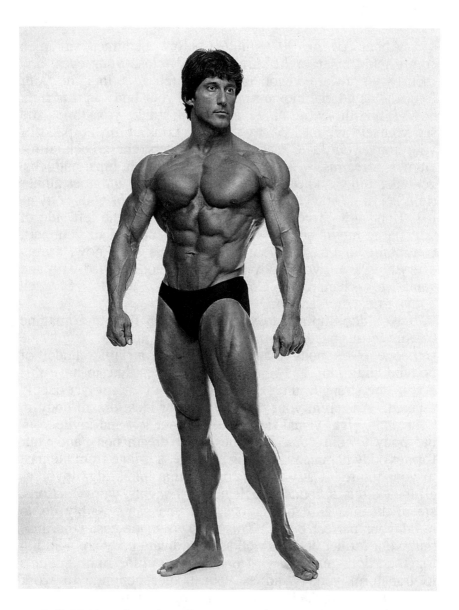

I SPEND HOURS VISUALIZING MY DREAM BODY

closer and closer, moving toward the middle of your bridge which is nearing completion.

Those areas on your former body you want to reduce, your dream body takes away.. Those areas you want to build, your dream body supplies the materials and gives you the exact instructions and messages on how to do it. This exchange continues until you meet your dream body at the top of the bridge in the middle . You look at each other and, realizing that you are exactly the same, you merge and become one. You have become your ideal self, your new perfect body.

What this visualization exercise does is put you in direct touch with the only body you ever experience. This isn't even your physical body, but your brain's representation of your physical body-- your BODY IMAGE-- you experience your brain's model of your body as if it were your body. This body image is what we experience anytime we feel embodied, whether it is in our physical body or when we are dreaming (6).

By practicing this visualization every night, the you in your dreams, your dream body, will begin to change. And as it changes, corresponding changes will occur in your physical body, since both are related to body image. By consciously changing your body image, you unconsciously change your real physical development.

As you persist, you will develop the ability to become conscious while you are dreaming and experience lucid dreams. With this comes the opportunity to take charge and direct your dream, and concurrent with this will come the ability to take charge and become more aware and in control of your waking life. And the next time you are dreaming, remember to recognize that you are dreaming. Since this is your dream, you can do what needs to be done to develop the body of your dreams!

"The body is our school, our lesson, our protagonist, our beloved enemy, our shadow, and anima/animus, the deep friend of our soul. Our

263

bodies, so much stuff of the world, so sensitive to our inner images, are much more changeable than we think, more fluid and spiritual more infused with light than we guess. Our bodies finally become the jumping off place into the higher realms, and may accompany us in some higher form into other worlds." (7)

THE PATH IS THE GOAL

As your body, mind, and speech become more aligned and congruent, synchronicity happens. This is the experience of meaningful coincidence in your life. Your thoughts and your words become real. You read, think, say, or see something symbolic and it happens in your life. As I trained for the 1979 Mr. Olympia I discovered the **Parable of the White Path**, which helped me understand my life's journey and gave me faith, certainty, and inspiration to persist in my training:

"Suppose there is a man who is traveling westward. On the way he suddenly confronts a river which is divided into two parts. One is a river of fire which flows to the south and the other is a river of water which flows to the north.

Each part is a hundred steps wide and unfathomably deep, extending endlessly to the south and to the north. Dividing the rivers of water and fire, there is a white path measuring four or five inches wide. This path is also one hundred steps long from the east bank to the west. The waves of the water splash and the flames of fire burn the path. The waves and flames alternate without ceasing.

He has already traveled far into the open plain where there is no one. Then there appear many bandits and beasts. Seeing him alone, they compete with each other to kill him. Afraid of death, he at once runs to the west. When he suddenly sees this great river, he says to himself, 'This river extends endlessly to the south and to the north. I see a white path in the middle which is extremely narrow.

'Although the two banks are close to each other, how can I get across? Undoubtably, I am bound to die this day. When I turn around to return, I see bandits and beasts coming closer and closer. If I try to run toward the south or the north, I see evil beasts and poisonous insects competing with each other in attacking me. If I seek the path to the west, there is, I am afraid, a danger of falling into the two rivers of water and fire.'

His horror at this moment is beyond expression. So he thinks to himself, 'If I turn back now, I shall die; If I stay I shall die; If I go forward, I shall die too. As I cannot escape death in any way, I would rather follow this path. **Since there is a path, it must be possible to cross.**'

As he is thinking thus, he suddenly hears a voice from the eastern bank urging him, 'You should determinedly follow this path. There will certainly be no danger of death. If you stay you will die.' Again, there is a person on the western bank, who calls, 'Come at once single-mindedly and right mindedly. I will protect you. Do not fear that you may fall into the calamities of water or fire.'

Since this person hears the urging voice on this bank and the calling from the other, he, with a determined mind, takes to the path and proceeds at once without doubt or fear. As he takes a step or two he hears the voices of the bandits on the eastern bank.

'Come back. The path is treacherous. You cannot cross it. Undoubtedly you are sure to die. We have no evil thought in pursuing you.' This person, though hearing many voices, does not even look back. As he proceeds straight on his way

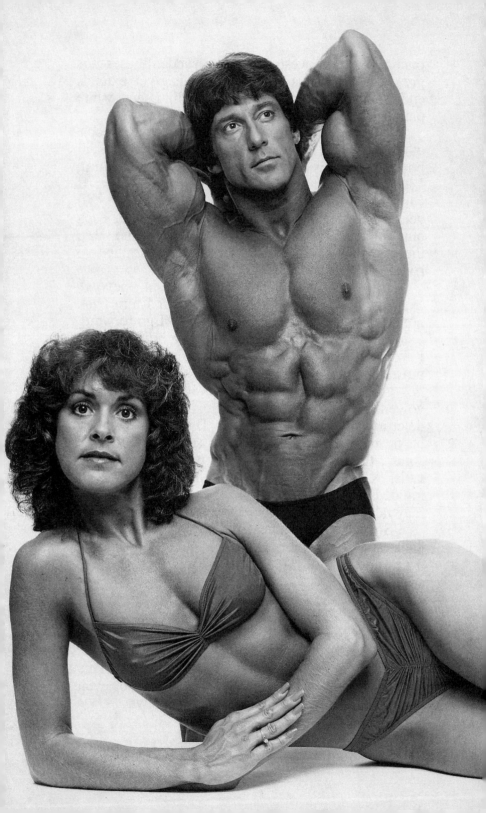

single-mindedly, he reaches the western bank in no time and is now free from all danger. There he meets his good friend, and his joy is endless." (8)

In order to reach the desired state and embrace a higher life, one must cross a river of greed and lust symbolized by water, and anger and hatred symbolized by fire. Raised in the human passions of greed and anger is your good mind containing your inner wish, goal, or purpose in life. Since the greed and anger are intense they are compared to water and fire. Since the good mind is weak, it is compared to the narrow white path. This path is in the middle and avoids the extremes. With a mind certain of success, concentrate on each step of the path, and you will reach your goal.

"One who determines to clean up the ocean is able, after a billion years, to clean up the ocean and to take treasures from the bottom of the ocean. If a person seeks the way, honestly, diligently, without giving up, he is able to reach the goal. Any kind of wish can be realized." (9)

THE PURPOSE OF THE BODY

As we mature, we can become more aware of our purpose in life, which is also the purpose of our body. Bodybuilding can lead to such self realization and character completion by helping us develop the ideal self that we would like to become. This ideal self is the embodiment of our true Inner, Larger, Higher Self, or Master within us who stays hidden until we reach the critical level of development by working on ourselves. A wholistic discipline encompassing our physical, mental, emotional, and spiritual nature, bodybuilding is a yoga of character completion. In the words of Sri Aurobindo:

"If our seeking is for a total perfection of the being, the physical part of it cannot be left aside; for the body is the material basis, the body is the instrument we have to use...life accomplishing its own spiritual transformation even here on earth in the conditions of the material universe. That cannot be unless the body too, undergoes a transformation, unless its action and functioning attain to a supreme capacity..." (10)

Our purpose as bodybuilders aspiring to become fully functioning human beings, is to develop the body to be a symbol of health and beauty, a vehicle fit for the journey that is our life. As long as the vehicle is maintained in good condition we will enjoy health and vigor and the journey will be fun and rewarding. This book is meant to be a guide toward this goal. I've made a map of my exploration, but this map is not the actual territory because I'm still traveling the path and midlife has rendered me farsighted. Practice the ideas and techniques I've given and you will fill in the details of your physical landscape with your own personal experience.

"I learned this, at least, by my experiment; that if one advances confidently in the direction of his dreams, and endeavors to live the life that he has imagined, he will meet with a success unexpected in common hours. He will put some things behind, will pass an invisible boundary; new, universal, and more liberal laws will begin to establish themselves around and within him; or the old laws be expanded, and interpreted in his favor in a more liberal sense, and he will live with the license of a higher order of beings. In proportion as he simplifies his life, the laws of the universe will appear less complex, and solitude will not be solitude, nor poverty poverty, nor weakness weakness. If you have built castles in the air, your work will not be lost; that is where they should be. Now put the foundations under them." (11)

You will be fabulously fit forever.

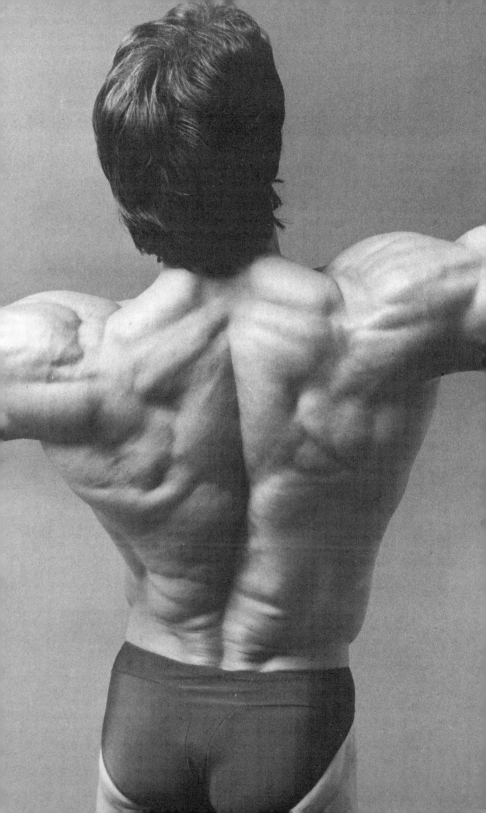

AFTERTHOUGHTS

A horseman from his point of vantage saw a poisonous snake slip down the throat of a sleeping man. The horseman realized that if the man were allowed to sleep the venom would surely kill him.

Accordingly, he lashed the sleeper until he was awake. Having no time to lose, he forced this man to a place where there were a number of rotten apples lying upon the ground and made him eat them. Then he made him drink large gulps of water from a stream.

All the while the man was trying to get away, crying: "What have I done, you enemy of humanity, that you should abuse me in this manner?" Finally when he was near to exhaustion, and dusk was falling, the man fell to the ground and vomited out the apples, the water, and the snake.

When he saw what had come out of him, he realized what had happened, and begged the forgiveness of the horseman. Then the man who was saved said: "If you had told me, I would have accepted your treatment with a good grace."

The horseman answered: "If I had told you, you would not have believed. Or you would have been paralysed by fright. Or run away. Or gone to sleep again, seeking forgetfulness. And there would not have been time."

Spurring his horse, the mysterious rider rode away.

Indries Shah (12)

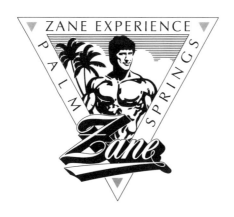

After retiring from bodybuilding competition, Christine and I opened Zane Haven, a bodybuilding learning center in Palm Springs, California. In the decade that followed, we trained thousands of men and women in the bodybuilding lifestyle. Although Zane Haven no longer exists, I have carried on the program in the format of the **Zane Experience**.

This book contains all the information formerly taught at Zane Haven plus new material that I teach in the Zane Experience. If you would like to work with me on a one-to-one basis in my private gym and experience the techniques in this book first hand, please feel free to contact me.

I will design a weight training, stretching, aerobic, nutritional, stress reduction, and motivational program just for you to help you get in the best shape of your life. I will give you my honest evaluation of your potential and teach you shortcuts that will save you years of costly mistakes.

Prior weight training experience is recommended but not essential. Familiarize yourself with the material in this book and you will get the most from working personally with me.

For more information write:

**ZANE EXPERIENCE
PO BOX 2031
PALM SPRINGS, CA 92263**
Phone 619-323-7486, FAX 619-323-2888

REFERENCES

INTRODUCTION

1. Neugarten, B.L. (1979). Time, Age, and the Life Cycle, in *American Journal of Psychiatry*, July, p. 887.

CHAPTER 1

1. Satir, V. (1976). *Making Contact*. Millbrae, Ca.: Celestial Arts.

2. Meatloaf, from the movie *Roadie*.

3. Hetherington, E., & Deur J. (1971). The effect of absence on child development. *Young Children*, 26, p. 233.

4. Tanner, J. (1970). Physical Growth, in *Carmichael's Manual of Child Psychology*, V.1.

5. Lowen, A. (1975). *Bioenergetics*. New York: Cowan, p. 119-120.

6. Hall, C. (1954). *A Primer of Freudian Psychology*. New York: Mentor Books.

7. Datan, N. (1980). Midas and other midlife crises. In *Midlife: Developmental and Clinical Issues*. New York: Brunner/Mazel, p. 3.

8. Hall, C.& Nordby, V. (1973). *A Primer of Jungian Psychology*. New York: Mentor Books.

9. Jung, C. in von Franz, M.L. (1974). *Shadow and Evil in Fairy Tales*. Dallas, Tx.: Spring Publ. p. 5.

10. Stevens W. (1954). Six Significant Landscapes. From Harmonium, published in *The Collected Poems of Wallace Stevens*. New York: Alfred Knopf. p. 74.

11. Ibid 8. p. 46.

12. Neugarten, B. (1979). Time Age, & the Life Cycle. *American Journal of Psychiatry*, July.

13. Evans W., & Rosenberg, I (1991). *Biomarkers*. New York: Simon & Schuster.

14. Murphy, M. (1992). *The Future of the Body*. Los Angeles: Tarcher. p. 425-431.

15. Ibid 14. P. 431.

16. Jung, C. (1930). The Stages of Life. *Collected Works*, 8, Bolligen Series, Princeton U. Press.

17. Dychtwald, K. (1989). *Age Wave*. Los Angeles: Tarcher.

18. Skinner, B.F. (1983). *Enjoy Old Age*. New York: Warner. p. 38-39, 146.

CHAPTER 2

1. Schwarzenegger, A. (1992). Address to National Press Club. *New Haven Register*, May 2, p. 21.

2. Jung, C. (1930). The Stages of Life. In *The Portable Jung*. New York: Penguin Books. p. 22.

3. Evans W. & Rosenberg, I. (1991). *Biomarkers*. New York: Simon & Schuster. A 12 week program of strength training with 60 and 70 year old men resulted in substantial strength increases with muscles that were larger and leaner with less fat in and around them. An 8 week study of 87 to 96 year old women confined to a nursing home tripled their muscles' strength and increased muscle size by 10 percent.

CHAPTER 3

1. Suzuki, S. (1970). *Zen Mind, Beginners Mind*. New York: Weatherhill, p. 21.

2. Shah, I. (1967). *Tales of the Dervishes*. Adapted from The Three Dervishes, p. 103-106. New York: Dutton.

3. Ebbinghaus, H. (1885). *Memory: A Contribution to Experimental Psychology*.

4. Anderson, J.R. (1976). *Language, Memory, and Thought*.

5. Anderson, B. (1980). *Stretching*. Bolinas, Ca: Shelter.

CHAPTER 4

1. Dooling, D.M. (1986). The Secret of the Wood. In *A Way of Working*. New York: Parabola Books.

2. Murphy, M. (1992). *The Future of the Body*. Los Angeles: Tarcher. p. 139. "The Taoist doctrine of wu wei, unblocked or unimpeded doing refers to such activity."

CHAPTER 5

1. Wallas, L. (1985). Adapted from Journey From a Frozen Land. In *Stories for the Third Ear*. New York: Norton & Co. p. 151-156.

2. Markus, H. & Nurius, P. (1986). Possible Selves. *American Psychologist*, 41, 9, p. 954-969.

3. Stevens, W. (1954). Theory. From Harmonium, published in *The Collected Poems of Wallace Stevens*, New York: Alfred Knopf. p. 86.

CHAPTER 6

1. Gurdfieff, G. (1950). Adapted from *All and Everything*. New York: Dutton & Co. p. 1192-1201.

CHAPTER 7

1. Von Franz, M.L. (1970). The Secret Church told in *Interpretations of Fairy Tales*. Dallas, Tx: Spring Publications, p. 105. "This tale shows that repressing the anima for conventional reasons results in psychic self-mutilation. If one gets too high up (up on the roof), one loses one's natural contact with the earth (the leg)."

2. Fitzgerald, L. (1991). Overtraining increases the susceptibility to infection. *International Journal of Sports Medicine*, 12:S5-S8. This research showed that after a single exhaustive exercise session there is temporary immune depression, with marked changes in lymphocytes in both well conditioned athletes as well as untrained people which lasts for several hours.

3. Easwaran, E. (1986) *The Dhammapada*. Nilgiri Press.

4. Aristotle. *Poetics*, p. 1457.

5. Nietzche, F. (1908). Ecce Homo. sec. 3. In *The Basic Writings of Nietzsche*. p. 757. New York: The Modern Library.

6. Zane, F. & Zane, C. (1986). *Zane Nutrition*. New York: Simon & Schuster.

7. Boorstein, S. (1985). Notes on right speech as a psychotherapeutic technique. *The Journal of Transpersonal Psychology*, 17(1), p. 47-56.

8. Moorman, C. (1985). *Talk Sense to Yourself*. Portage, Mi.: Personal Power Press.

9. *Dorland's Illustrated Medical Dictionary* (1985). Philadelphia: W.B. Saunders Co., p. 716. According to the Arndt-Schulz Law, "Weak stimuli increase physiologic activity and very strong stimuli inhibit or abolish activity". An injury to muscle decreases adenosine triphosphate (ATP), causing spasm which in turn decreases oxygen and nutrient supply to cells and results in accumulation of metabolic waste products. Microcurrent stimulation replenishes ATP in injured tissues and increases membrane active transport which allows nutrients to flow into cells as waste products are removed. This increase in ATP generation and membrane transport allows enhanced protein synthesis and promotes formation of healthy tissue.

10. La Berge, S. (1985). *Lucid Dreaming*. New York: Ballantine Books. Lucid dreaming is conscious awarness during the dream state. LaBerge claims that by controlling your dream life you can change the quality of your waking life. Consequently, mental and physical health are enhanced through the healing power of the unconscious mind.

CHAPTER 8

1. Saito, G. & Sweany, J. (1977) translators. Adapted from *Shout of Buddha: Writings of Haya Akegarasu*. Chicago: Orchid Press. p. 10-15.

2. Metzner, R. (1980). Ten classical metaphors of self-transformation. *Journal of Transpersonal Psychology*, 12, 1, p. 59-60.

3. Wurtman, R., & Wurtman, J. (1989). Carbohydrates and Depression. *Scientific American*, January.

4. Pierpaoli, W. (1988). Melatonin extends rat lives. *Brain/Mind Bulletin*, 13, 9, June, p. 1,8. It was found that the addition of melatonin to the night time drinking water of mice improved performance, delayed symptoms of aging, and increased their lifespan by 20 percent.

5. Liberman, J. (1991). *Light: Medicine of the Future*. Santa Fe, N.M.: Bear Publishing Co.

6. Ibid 5. p. 151.

CHAPTER 9

1. Robinson, J., translator (1979). Adapted from Sarvabhaksa in *Buddha's Lions*. Berkeley, Ca.: Dharma Publishing. p. 231-2.

2. Walford, R. (1983). *Maximum Life Span*. New York: Avon. p.96.

3. *Recommended Dietary Allowances* (1980). Washington D.C.: National Academy of Sciences.

4. Rudman, D. et al (1990). Effects of human growth hormone in men over 60 years old. *New England Journal of Medicine*, p. 323, 1, July.

5. Zane, F. & Zane, C. (1986). *Zane Nutrition*. New York: Simon & Schuster.

6. Netzer, C. (1992). *The Corinne T. Netzer Encyclopedia of Food Values*. New York: Dell.

7. Silverman, M. (1976). *The Drugging of the Americas*. Berkeley, Ca.: University of California Press.

8. Alen, M., et. al (1987). Androgenic-anabolic steroid effects on serum thyroid, pituitary, and steroid hormones in athletes. *American Journal of Sports Medicine*. 15(4), July-August: p. 357-361.

9. Friedman, M. et. al (1958). Changes in serum cholesterol and blood clotting time in men subject to cyclic variation of occupational stress. *Circulation*, 17, p. 852-861.

10. van Doomen, L., & Orlebeke, K. (1982). Stress, personality, and serum cholesterol level. *Journal of Human Stress*, 8, p. 24-29.

11. Metaform Technically Advanced Nutrition Packets are available in both chocolate and original flavors and are available at GNC Stores. Distributed by Great American Nutrition, Salt Lake City, Utah.

12. Zane, C. (1993). *The Zane Nutrition Cookbook*. Zananda, Inc., PO Box 2031, Palm Springs, Ca. 92263.

CHAPTER 10

1. Bentov, I. (1977). *Stalking the Wild Pendulum*. Rochester, Vt.: Destiny Books. p. 25.

2. Benson, H. (1975). *The Relaxation Response*. New York: Avon. p. 178.

3. Selye, H. (1956). *The Stress of Life*. New York: McGraw Hill. p. vii.

4. Garwood, et. al. (1982). Autonomic nervous system function and aging: Response specificity. *Psychophysiology*, 19, p. 378-385. It was found that with men ages 30 to 80, the older the subjects, the more consistent they were in their physiological response to a variety of stressors.

5. Ibid 1, p. 70.

6. Murphy, M. (1992). *The Future of the Body*. Los Angeles: Jeremy Tarcher. p. 603-610. Murphy has collected hundreds of scientific references on the benefits of meditation.

7. Wallace, R.K. (1970). Physiological effects of transcendental meditation. *Science*, p. 166. It was discovered that the decrease in the volume of oxygen consumed during meditation was 20 percent below base rate.

8. Pitts, F. (1969). The biochemistry of anxiety. *Scientific American*, February.

9. Ibid 7.

10. Goleman, D. (1971). Meditation as meta-therapy. *Journal of Transpersonal Psychology*, 1, p. 1-25.

11. Goleman, D. (1991). Tibetan and Western Models of Mental Health, in *MindScience*. Boston: Wisdom Pulications, p. 92-95. Copyright Mind/Body Medical Institute Inc. and Tibet House New York Inc. 1991, Reprinted from *MindScience* with permission of Wisdom Publications, 361 Newbury St., Boston, Massachusetts USA.

12. Lewis, J. (1970). Semantic processing of unattended messages using dichotic listening. *Journal of Experimental Psychology*, 85, p. 225-228.

13. Forster, P.M. & Govier, E. (1978). Discrimination without awareness? *Quarterly Journal of Experimental Psychology*, 30, p. 282-95.

14. Nielsen, S.L. & Sarason, I.G. (1981). Emotion, personality, and selective attention. *Journal of Personality and Social Psychology*, 41(5), p. 945-960.

15. Kurtz, R.S. (1986). Subliminal messages for weight loss. *Masters Abstracts*, 26(1), p. 159.

16. Russell, T.G. (1989). The effect of subliminal auditory messages upon academic achievement. *Dissertation Abstracts International*, 50/06-B, p. 2609.

17. Nordstrom, R.R. (1980). The placebo effect, subliminal perception, and hypnotic induction. *Hypnosis Quarterly*, 23(3). p. 9-12.

18. Zane, F. (1990). *The Effects of Dichotic Listening on Aerobic Performance.* Western Psychological Association, Los Angeles, April. Since a style of awareness that divides the attention may be conducive to aerobic exercise performance, dichotic audio tapes can also be used to help people do stationary aerobic exercise for longer periods of time. The results of research I completed to earn a Master's Degree in Experimental Psychology showed that people exercised significantly longer at target pulse rate and burned more calories when they listened to dichotic audio tapes. The high degree of cognitive complexity of the dichotic tape helped transform the boring repetitive stationary aerobic exercise into a more interesting activity and prevent performance decrement.

19. Hutchison, M. (1990). *Consciousness Technology.* Sausalito, Ca.

20. Yerkes, R. & Dodson, J. (1908). The relation of strength of stimulus to rapidity of habit formation. *Journal of Comparative Neurology & Psychology*, 18, p. 459-482.

21. Jacobson, E. (1929). *Progressive Relaxation.* Chicago: University of Chicago Press.

22. Tart, C. (1990). Adapting Eastern spiritual teachings to Western culture. *Journal of Transpersonal Psychology*, 22, p. 2.

23. Zane, F. (1993). *Fabulously Fit Forever.* Palm Springs: Zananda, Inc. Brain waves represent the electrical patterns of millions of neurons or brain cells. The four major categories of brain wave frequencies (measured in

cycles per second or hz.) are beta (13 to 30 hz), the brain wave of eyes open conscious outward awareness; alpha (8 to 12 hz), the relaxed eyes closed non-drowsy tranquil brain wave of inward awareness and meditation; theta (4 to 7 hz) the drowsy brain wave of visual imagery, creativity, and advanced meditators; and delta (0.5 to 3 hz), the slowest brain wave of deep dreamless sleep and growth hormone secretion.

24. My mind gym consists of a *Brainware 200* Mind/Body Exercise System (*B-200*) whose microprocessor diffuses light waves over my closed eyelids, creating a pleasant kaleidoscopic light show. The headset has light screen plus earphones built in which adds rhythmic synchronized ocean waves to the sounds of the Dichotic or Beat Frequency Audio Cassettes I play thru the *B-200* with the stereo patchcord. I adjust brightness and volume with the user friendly dials.

Before workouts, I use *B-200* programs that start at a low frequency (3 to 6 hz) and sweep gradually upward to a target frequency (14 to 18 hz), staying there for the duration of the program until it sweeps down to the end frequency of 13 hz, bringing me out of the session at low beta/ high alpha waves. I feel energized and alert when I start my workout. I generally make the length of these programs 15 to 20 minutes. I like to use my tapes 1, 5, 15, 24, and 25 with these programs.

After workouts, I use *B-200* programs that start at 20 hz and sweep down to 10, 11, or 12 hz for visualization; 7, 8, or 9 hz for meditation; and 4, 5, or 6 hz for deep rest. I end these programs at 13 hz by engaging the automatic frequency return and do them for 20 to 30 minutes. Before bcd, I start at 20 hz and end at 2 or 3 hz with a program length of 15 to 25 minutes. I use my tapes 2, 4, 6, 9, 12, 13, 14, 16, 20, 21, 22, 23, & 27 with these programs.

I often use manual control on the *B-200* set at 11 hz and either move upward to 18 hz for energizing or downward to 7 hz for deep meditation. I often perform the meditation on breathing (see page 193) in time to the synchronized waves from the *B-200*, or I use these audio tapes with the manual program for motivation: 3, 6, 7, 8, 10, 11, 23, 24, 25, & 26. The length of these programs is 20 or 25 minutes.

WARNING: People who are subject to epilepsy, seizures, heart disorders or any abnormal neurological condition should NOT use the *Brainware 200* without first consulting a medical professional.

25. Morton, L. & Kershner, J. (1984). Negative air ionization improves memory and attention in learning disabled and mentally retarded children. *Journal of Abnormal Child Psychology*, June, V. 12(2), p. 353-365. The mechanism is believed to involve the action of negative ions on the neurotransmitter serotonin.

26. Patten, L. (1988). *Biocircuits*. Kramer: Tiburon, Ca.

27. Isaacs, J. (1991). The Biocircuit Study: Evidence for Relaxation Effects, in *Tools for Exploration*, San Rafael, Ca.: Professional Technologies, Inc.

28. Shapiro, C.M. et. al. (1981). Slow wave sleep: a recovery period after exercise. *Science*, 214, p. 1253-54. This study examined the sleep of trained athletes who competed in a 57 mile marathon. Slow wave sleep increased 40 and 45 percent in the two nights following the race, whereas total amount of sleep increased only 18 and 27 percent respectively. The participants also spent less time in REM sleep these same two nights.

29. Moldofsky, H. & Scarisbrick, P. (1976). Induction of neuroasthenic musculoskeletal pain syndrome by selective sleep stage deprivation. *Psychosomatic Medicine*, 38, p. 35-44.

30. Easwaran, E. (1977). *Formulas for Transformation*. Petaluma, Ca.: Nilgiri Press. p. 214-215.

CHAPTER 11

1. Orage, A.R. *On Love*. New York: Samuel Weiser.

2. Lee, J. A. (1974). Styles of loving. *Psychology Today*. 8(5), p. 43-51.

3. Gaines, C. & Butler, G. (1974). *Pumping Iron*. New York: Simon & Schuster, p. 48.

4. Berscheid, E. & Walster, E. (1974). Physical attractiveness. *Advances in Experimental Social Psychology*, 7, p. 157-215.

5. Schacter, S. (1964). The interaction of cognitive and physiological determinants of emotional state. In L. Berkowitz (Ed.), *Advances in Experimental Social Psychology*. V. 1, New York: Academic Press.
6. White, G.L., et. al. (1981). Passionate love and the misattribution of arousal. Journal of Personality and Social Psychology, 41, p. 56-62.

7. Hall, C.S. (1954). *A Primer of Freudian Psychology*. New York: Mentor Books.

8. Maslow, A.H. (1968). *Toward a Psychology of Being*. Princeton, N.J.: Van Nostrand.

9. Fromm, E. (1956). *The Art of Loving*. New York: Harper & Row.

CHAPTER 12

1. Guardini, R. (1954). The Spiritual Body. In *The Last Things*. London: Burns & Oates. p. 61.

2. Stevens, W. (1954). Hymn from a watermelon patch. From Harmonium, published in *The Collected Poems of Wallace Stevens*. p.89

3. Chinmoy, S. (1992). *Sayings of Sri Chinmoy*. New York: Manifestation Glow Press.

4. Allen, J. (1970). *As a Man Thinketh*. New York: National Colorgraphics, p. 23-24.

5. Rhode, E. (1893). *Psyche*. Liepzig.

6. La Berge, S. & Rheingold, H. (1990). *Exploring the World of Lucid Dreaming*. New York: Ballantine. I highly recommend this book to those interested in becoming proficient at lucid dreaming.

7. Conger, J. (1988). *Jung & Reich: The Body as Shadow*. Berkeley, Ca.: North Atlantic Books. p. 189.

8. Shonin, S. (1978). Teaching, Practice, Faith, & Enlightenment. In *Shinshu Seiten*. Buddhist Churches of America, 1710 Octavia Street, San Francisco, Ca 94109. p. 95-98.

9. Saito, G. & Sweeny, J. (1977). trans. *Shout of Buddha: Writings of Haya Akegarasu*. Chicago: Orchid Press. p. 54.

10. Aurobindo, S. (1971). *The Mind of Light*. New York: Dutton, p. 34.

11. Thoreau, H. D. (1854). Walden. in *Walden and Other Writngs by Henry David Thoreau*, ed. Krutch, J. W., 1962. New York: Bantam. P. 343.

12. Shah I. (1970). The Horseman and the Snake, in *Tales of the Dervishes*. New York: Dutton. P. 140-141.

BODYBUILDING DIARY

DREAM WORK: Record whatever you can remember of your dream, your feelings, and finish the dream the way you want it to end.

FOOD JOURNAL: Write your food, amount in ounces, time eaten, grams of nutritents, calories, & calories from fat.

FOOD OUNCES TIME PROTEIN FAT CARB CALORIES FAT CAL.

VISUAL REHEARSAL: Before your workout, visualize your training session, see yourself doing reps in great form on each exercise.

TRAINING ROUTINE: Write down each exercise, sets, reps, and weight used and stretches right after you do them or after you finish training.

EXERCISES	SETS	REPS/WEIGHT	STRETCH

DEEP RELAXATION: After your workout, meditate, listen to audio tapes, use your *Brainware 200* Mind/Body Training System, or lie down and close your eyes for 20 minutes and repeat your power phrase.

DREAM BODY VISUALIZATION: Right before bedtime, close your eyes and visualize your ideal body (as in Chapter 12).

THE WORKOUTS

All the routines in the book are listed here. Use this form as your workout journal.

KID'S FULL BODY ROUTINE

Barbell Clean and Press & Doorway Stretch
Barbell Bent Forward Row & 2 Arm Lat Stretch
Barbell Bench Press & Doorway Stretch
Dumb bell Curl & Arms Back Stretch
Sit-up & 1 Leg Up Stretch
Front Squat & 1 Leg Back Stretch
Calf Raise & Calf Stretch

SENIOR'S ROUTINE

Leg Extension & 1 Leg Back Stretch
Leg Curl & 1 Leg Up Stretch
Standing Calf Raise & Calf Stretch
Lying Knee-in
Front Pulldown & 2 Arm Lat Stretch
Pec Deck & Doorway Stretch
1 Arm Dumb bell Side Raise & I Arm Shoulder Stretch
1 Arm Dumb bell Curl & Pronated Arms Back Stretch
1 Arm Dumb bell Kickback & Arms Back Stretch

BEGINNER'S FULL BODY ROUTINE

Incline Dumb bell Press & Doorway Stretch

One Arm Dumb bell Row & 2 arm Lat Stretch

Dumb bell fly & Doorway Stretch

Dumb bell Pullover & 1 Arm Shoulder Stretch

Dumb bell Rear Deltoid Raise & Rear Delt Stretch

Dumb bell Kickback & Arms Back Stretch

Dumb bell Curls & Pronated Arms Back Stretch

Dumb bell Side Raise & 1 Arm Shoulder Stretch

Barbell Reverse Curl & Pronated Arms back Stretch

Erect Front Squat & 1 Leg Back Stretch

Hyperextension & 1 Leg Up Stretch

One Legged Calf Raise & Calf Stretch

Knee in

Seated Twist

Incline Partial Situp

UPPER BODY / LOWER BODY SPLIT ROUTINE

DAY 1: UPPER BODY

75 Degree Incline DB Press & Doorway Stretch
Front Pulldown & 2 Arm Lat Stretch
30 Degree Incline DB Press & Doorway Stretch
DB Rear Delt Raise & Rear Delt Stretch
DB Fly & Doorway Stretch
DB Pullover & 1 Arm Shoulder Stretch
Seated Low Cable Row & 2 Arm Lat Stretch
DB Kickback & Arms Back Stretch
Face Down Incline DB Curl & Pronated arms back stretch
DB Side Raise & 1 Arm Shoulder Stretch
Barbell Reverse Curl & Pronated Arms Back Stretch
Knee in
Seated Twist
Incline Partial Sit-up
Rowing Ergometer or Airdyne

DAY 2: LOWER BODY

Leg Extension & One Leg Back Stretch
Leg Curl & One Leg Up Stretch
Good Morning Exercise & One Leg Up Stretch
Erect Squat & One Leg Back Stretch
Lunge & One Leg Up Stretch
Side Leg Raise with Ankle Weights
Standing Calf Raise & Calf Stretch
Donkey Calf Raise & Calf Stretch
Leg Raise
Seated Twist
Crunches

2 WAY SPLIT ROUTINE FOR WEIGHT LOSS

DAY 1: FULL BODY

30 Degree Incline DB Press & Doorway Stretch
75 Degree Incline DB Press & Doorway Stretch
DB Fly & Doorway Stretch
DB Pullover & 1 Arm Lat Stretch
Front Pulldown & 2 Arm Lat Stretch
DB Bent Over Row & 2 Arm Lat Stretch
DB Kickback & Arms Back Stretch
Face Down Incline DB Curl & Pronated Arms Back Stretch
DB Side Raise & Rear Delt Stretch
DB Rear Delt Raise & Rear Delt Stretch
Leg Raise
Incline Partial Situp
Seated Twist
Leg Curl & 1 Leg Up Stretch
Leg Extension & 1 Leg Back Stretch
Lunge & 1 Leg Up Stretch
Stairclimber & 1 Leg Back Stretch

DAY 2: LOWER BODY

Warmup on Stationary Bike
Leg Extension & 1 Leg Back Stretch
Leg Curl & 1 Leg Up Stretch
Good Morning Exercise & 1 Leg Up Stretch
Standing Calf Raise & Calf Stretch
Sissy Squat & 1 Leg Back Stretch
Side Leg Raise with ankle weights
Rear Leg Raise with ankle weights
Seated Twist
Knee Ups
Crunches
Treadmill

BEGINNING AB-AEROBICS

Leg Raise

Rowing Machine

Seated Twist

Stairclimber

Crunches

Stationary Bike

ADVANCED AB-AEROBICS

Incline Knee up

Rowing Machine

Incline Partial Situp

Stationary Bike

Flat Leg Raise

Stairclimber

Hyperextension

Treadmill

Seated Twist

Crunches

Airdyne

THE 3 WAY SPLIT ROUTINE

DAY 1: BACK, BICEPS, FOREARMS

BACK

Front Pulldown & 2 Arm Lat Stretch

Seated Low Cable Row & 2 Arm Lat Stretch

Bent Over DB Upright Row & 2 Arm Lat Stretch

1 Arm DB Row & 1 Arm Lat Stretch

BICEPS

Alternate DB Curl & Pronated Arms Back Stretch

Face Down Incline DB Curl & same stretch

Incline DB Curl & same stretch

FOREARMS

BB Reverse Curl & Pronated Arms Back Stretch

BB Wrist Curl & same stretch

ABDOMINALS   AEROBICS: Rowing

Leg Raise

Crunches

Seated Twist

Hyperextension

DAY 2: THIGHS & CALVES

THIGHS

>Leg Extension & 1 Leg Back Stretch

>Leg Curl & 1 Leg Up Stretch

>Erect Squat & 1 Leg Up Stretch

>Lunge & 1 Leg Up Stretch

>Stairclimber

CALVES

>Standing Calf Raise & Calf Stretch

>Seated Calf Raise & same stretch

>Donkey Calf Raise & same stretch

ABDOMINALS (super-setted)

>Leg Raise
>Crunches

>Knee-ups
>Partial Incline Situp

>Seated Twist
>One Arm Cable Crunch

>Hyperextension

AEROBICS: Stationary Bike

DAY 3: CHEST, SHOULDERS, TRICEPS

CHEST

    30 Degree Incline DB Press & Doorway Stretch

    75 Degree Incline DB Press & Doorway Stretch

    or Front Press on Overhead Press Machine

    DB Fly & Doorway Stretch

    DB Pullover & 1 Arm Shoulder Stretch

TRICEPS

    Pressdown or DB Kickback & Arms Back Stretch

    Close Grip Bench & Arms Back Stretch

    1 Arm DB Extension & 1 Arm Shoulder Stretch

SHOULDERS

    Bent Over DB Rear Delt Raise & Rear Delt Str.

    1 Arm DB Side Raise & Rear Delt Stretch

ABDOMINALS   AEROBICS: airdyne

                                  or rowing

    Leg Raise

    Crunches

    Seated Twist

    Hyperextension

THE ADVANCED 3 WAY SPLIT ROUTINE

DAY 1 - BACK, BICEPS, FOREARMS

BACK (super-setted)

> Front Pulldown
> Cable Crossover Behind Neck & 2 arm lat stretch
>
> Seated Low Cable Row
> Bent Over Rear Cable Raise & 2 arm lat stretch
>
> 1 Arm DB Row
> 1 Arm Cable Row & 1 arm lat stretch

BICEPS (super-setted)

> Bistar Curl *
> DB Concentration Curl **
>
> Face Down Incline DB Curl
> Preacher Cable Curl & pronated arms back str.

FOREARMS (tri-setted)

> BB Reverse Wrist Curl
> Barbell Wrist Curl
> Hand Gripper & pronated arms back stretch

ABDOMINALS (at end of workout or later in the day)

AEROBICS (Rowing at end of workout or later in the day)

note: * If you don't have Bistars, do: Seated 1 Arm DB Curl
  ** super-setted with One Arm DB Concentration Curl

DAY 2 - CALVES, THIGHS

ABDOMINALS: Can be done at beginning of workout or later in the day

Pulley Knee In

Incline Leg Raise
Abdominal Crunch

Flat Leg Raise
Two Arm Cable Crunch

Seated Twist
1 Arm Cable Crunch

Hyperextension

CALVES (tri-setted)

Standing Calf Raise
Seated Calf Raise
Incline Calf Raise on *Soloflex Rockit* & calf stretch

THIGHS (super-setted)

Standing One Leg Curl
Hip Machine & 1 leg up stretch

Leg Extension & 1 leg back stretch
Leg Curl & 1 leg up stretch

Leg Blaster Squat
Stairclimber

AEROBICS: Stationary bike or treadmill at end of workout or later in the day

DAY 3 - CHEST, SHOULDERS, TRICEPS

CHEST/ FRONT DELTS (super-setted)

>   30 Degree Incline DB Press
>   Cable Crossover & doorway stretch
>
>   Pec Deck
>   Front Press Machine & doorway stretch
>
>   Dip Machine
>   Rear Delt Machine & doorway stretch
>
>   DB Pullover
>   Stiff Arm Pulldown & 1 arm shoulder stretch

SHOULDERS/ TRICEPS (super-setted)

>   1 Arm DB Tricep Extension
>   Bistar 1 Arm Side Raise * & 1 arm shoulder stretch
>
>   Triceps Pressdown
>   Pronated DB Side Raise & rear delt stretch
>
>   1 Arm Cable Kickback
>   1 Arm Side Cable Raise & arms back stretch

ABDOMINALS - Do at end of workout or later in the day

AEROBICS
>   Rowing or stationary bike at end of workout or later in the day.

* Or 1 arm DB side raise

BODYPART EXERCISE INDEX

Although each of the following exercises work more than a single bodypart, each exercise is listed under the main bodypart is effects with pages where it is found in the text.

BACK   **STRETCHES:** 53-56

BB Clean & Press - 34
Bent Forward Row - 35, 128
Front Pulldown - 69, 84, 103, 105, 128, 236
DB Pullover -59, 71, 84, 120, 122, 128, 242
Hyperextension -62, 95, 126, 127, 132, 245
Seated Low Cable Row -71, 103, 105, 128, 236
Concept II Rowing Ergometer - 94, 95, 96, 135
Bent Over DB Upright Row - 103, 106
One Arm DB Row - 59, 85, 103, 106, 128, 237
1 Arm Cable Row - 128, 237
Wide Grip Chins - 128
T Bar Row - 128
Cable Crossover Behind Neck - 236
Seated Machine Row - 131
Good Morning Exercise - 74,90
Bent Over Rear Cable Raise - 236

BICEPS

DB Curl (2 arm) - 35, 60
One Arm DB Curl - 41
Face Down (75 degree) Incline DB Curl - 72, 85, 103, 108, 238
Alternate DB Curl - 60, 103, 107
Incline DB Curl (45 degree) - 103, 108
Preacher Cable Curl - 238
Bistar Curl - 237
DB Concentration Curl - 237

FOREARMS

BB Reverse Curl - 61, 72, 103, 109
BB Wrist Curl - 103, 110, 238
Hand Gripper - 238
Reverse Wrist Curl - 238

THIGHS

Front Squat - 36, 61, 75
Leg Extension - 39, 74, 88, 89, 112, 113, 130, 240
Leg Curl - 39, 74, 87, 89, 112, 114, 130, 240
Erect Squat with Leg Blaster - 112, 116, 128, 130, 240
Good Morning Exercise - 74, 90
Lunge - 75, 88, 112, 117
Side Leg Raise - 75, 91
Treadmill - 92, 95, 96, 134
Stairclimber - 88, 95, 96, 112, 118, 134, 240
Stationary Bike - 89, 95, 96, 134
Sissy Squat - 90
Rear Leg Raise - 91
Barbell Squat - 115, 128
Leg Press - 128
Hip Machine - 240
Standing One Leg Curl - 239
Airdyne - 95, 96, 135

CALVES

Calf Raise - 36
One Legged Calf Raise - 62
Standing Calf Raise - 40, 76, 90, 112, 118, 128, 130, 239
Donkey Calf Raise - 76, 112, 119, 128
Seated Calf Raise - 112, 119, 239
Incline Calf Raise - 239
Treadmill, Stairclimber, Stationary Bike - (see Thighs)

CHEST

BB Bench Press - 35, 128
Pec Deck - 41, 128, 241
30 Degree Incline DB Press - 58, 70, 83, 120, 128, 240
DB Fly - 59, 70, 84, 120, 122, 128
DB Pullover - 59, 71, 84, 120, 122, 128, 242
Dip Machine - 128, 241
Incline Press Machine - 128
Vertical Bench Press Machine - 128
Cable Crossover - 240
Stiff Arm Pulldown (or serratus lever) - 242
Pullover Machine - 128

SHOULDERS

BB Clean & Press - 34
One Arm DB Side Raise - 41
Bistar Side Raise - 242
DB Side Raise (2 Arms) - 61, 72, 86, 125, 128
Pronated DB Side Raise - 243
DB Rear Deltoid Raise (Bent Over) - 60, 70, 86, 120, 125, 128
75 Degree Incline DB Press - 69, 83, 120, 121, 128
Machine Front Press - 120, 128, 241
Lateral Raise Machine - 128
Rear Delt Machine (or Nautilus Torso Row) - 128, 242
Dip Machine - 128, 241
1 Arm Side Cable Raise - 243
Bent Over Rear Cable Raise - 236

TRICEPS

One Arm DB Kickback - 42
DB Kickback (2 Arm) - 60, 71, 85
One Arm Cable Kickback - 243
Close Grip Bench Press - 120, 123
Dip Machine - 128, 241
Pressdown - 120, 123, 243
One Arm DB Extension - 120, 124, 242

ABDOMINALS

Situp - 36, 128
Lying Knee-in - 40, 95
Knee in - 62, 73
Incline Partial Situp - 63, 73, 87, 95, 127
Seated Twist - 63, 73, 77, 87, 91, 94, 95, 127, 128, 245
Crunches - 77, 92, 95, 127, 244
Knee-ups - 92, 127, 244
Incline Leg Raise - 245
Leg Raise - 76, 86, 94, 95, 127
One Arm Cable Crunch - 245
2 Arm Cable Crunch - 245
Pulley Knee in - 244

BRAIN

Brainware 200 Mind/Body Exercise System - 203, 304
Dichotic Audio Tapes - 198, 307
Bio-circuit - 209

ACKNOWLEDGEMENTS/PICTURE CREDITS:

I wish to thank my wife Christine Zane, whose suggestion and support made this book possible and whose drawings grace these pages.

John White for his ideas in organizing this material.

Abakash of Manifestation Glow for printing this book.

Joe Weider for providing the opportunity to express the ideas that appear in these pages in *Muscle & Fitness Magazine*.

The photographers whose photos appear on these pages:

CHRISTINE ZANE: 27, 32,34-36, 39-42, 53-56, 59 TOP & BOTTOM, 60 TOP & BOT, 61 TOP & MIDDLE, 63 TOP, 66, 69 BOT, 70 MID, 71 TOP & MID, 72 MID & BOT, 77, 83 BOT, 85 TOP, 86 TOP & MID, 88 BOT, 89 TOP, 92 MID, 94, 105, 106, 107, 108 BOT, 109, 110, 115, 118 TOP, 119 TOP, 121, 122 BOT, 125, 134 TOP & BOT, 136, 159, 176, 188, 203, 222, 225, 237 TOP, 238 TOP & MID, 240 BOT, 241 MID & BOT, 242 MID, 243 BOT, 250 LEFT, 251 TOP RT & BOT LT, 300, 308, 316.

ART ZELLER: 20, 23, 44, 110, 164, 192, 220, 235, 246, 250 RT, 251 BOT RT, 252 RT, 256, 304.

MIKE NEVEUX: 7, 63 BOT, 252 LT, 253.

JACK MITCHELL: 48, 49, 58, 63 MID & BOT, 64, 69 TOP 70 TOP, 73 TOP, 73 MID, 75 MID, 76 TOP & MID, 80, 83 TOP, 84 BOT, 85 TOP & MID, 86 TOP & MID, 87 MID & BOT, 88 TOP & MID, 90 MID, 91 BOT, 92 TOP, 99, 111, 119 BOT, 120, 123 BOT, 124, 146, 218, 262, 266, 300.

KENN DUNCAN: 59 MID, 60 MID, 61 BOT, 70 BOT, 71 BOT, 74 BOT, 75 TOP & BOT, 76 BOT, 84 TOP & MID, 86 BOT, 90 TOP & BOT, 91 TOP & MID, 104, 122 TOP, 156, 213, 214, 237 BOT, 248, 269, 310.

RALPH DeHAAN: 62 TOP, 63 MID, 72 TOP, 73 BOT, 74 TOP & MID, 85 BOT, 87 TOP, 89 MID & BOT, 92 BOT, 108 TOP, 113, 114, 116, 117, 118 BOT, 123 TOP, 126, 130, 131 TOP & BOT, 132, 134, 236, 237, 238, 249 TOP, 241, TOP, 242 TOP & BOT, 243 TOP & MID, 245, BACK COVER.

BILL DOBBINS: FRONT COVER, 31, 100, 187, 302.

JOHN BALIK: 50, 168, 251 TOP LT.   **BOB GARDNER** - 306, 333.

ROBERT REIFF - 130, 131, 133, 135, 203, 239 TOP, 314, 315, 324, 326.

FRANK ZANE: 43, 155.

FLASHBACKS

GREAT WORKOUTS FROM THE PAST

I often think of the elaborate training programs I did at the height of my competitive career. When I look back through my training journals from the 1970's and early 1980's, I'm amazed at the amount of work I did in these training sessions. Here is an example of a workout I did in preparing for the 1979 Mr. Olympia. This chest, shoulder, triceps workout took place 8:30 to 10:30 pm September 3, 1979, one month before the Mr. Olympia Contest. Christine and I arrived at Gold's Gym, which was then located on 2nd Street in Santa Monica, a little before closing time and trained together for two hours. We were both very strong: Christine deadlifted 270 for 2 reps and I used heavy weights on all my exercises. It took a long time to wind down from this late workout and we were very tired the next morning. Christine did most of the exercises with me but with lighter weights. Here's the workout taken from my training journal:

Chest
    Bench Press - 135pounds/10 reps, 185/10, 235/10, 260/8, 280/5, 300/2 (slow negatives)
    45 Degree Incline DB Press - 65s/10, 75s/10, 85s/8, 95s/6
    Dips on Nautilus Multi-Machine - 20/10, 30/9, 40/8, 50/6

Delts
    Front Press Universal Machine - 120/10, 135/8, 145/7, 60/5
    1 DB Front Raise - 55/12, 60/11, 65/10
    Nautilus Side Raise Machine - 80/12, 90/11, 100/10, 110/9
    Nautilus Torso Row (rear delts)- 60/10 reps, 4sets
    1 Arm Side Cable Raise - 15/10 - 3 non-stop sets
                                    with each arm

Back to Chest again
    Nautilus 2 Way Chest Machine:
    Pec Deck - 80/12, 90/11, 100/10 super-setted with
    Decline Press - 90/10, 100/10

    Cable Crossover - 60/12, 70/11, 80/10
    DB Pullover - 85, 95, 100, 110 for 10 reps

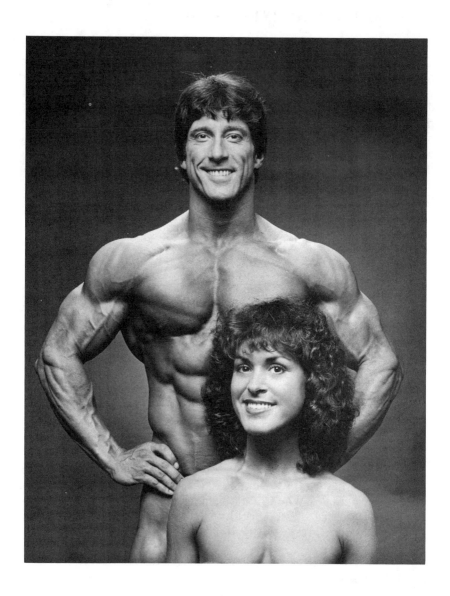

Triceps
- 1 Arm DB Extension - 35/10, 40/8, 45/7, 50/6
- Close Grip Bench Press on Smith Machine - 135/10, 155/8, 175/6
- Pressdown - 80/12, 90/11, 100/10, 110/8

Abs
- Hanging Knee Up - 3 sets of 50 reps super setted with
- Crunches - 3 sets of 50 reps
- 1 Arm Cable Crunch - 3 sets 25 reps each arm with 80 pounds
- Hyperextension - 2 sets of 25 reps

This workout totals 26 sets for chest, 18 sets for deltoids, and 11 sets for triceps. Total amount of sets for the workout is 55, as compared to approximately 35 sets in my current workout. In 1979 I used 15 exercises (not counting ab work), while in 1995, I'm still doing 15 exercises in a workout. This is the same amount of exercises but fewer total sets, and twice as much abdominal work. Why the difference?

It's not that I'm putting any less importance on training. The main effect of my workouts now as compared to then is that I am still getting sore from these training sessions. It would be foolish to try to do more sets with heavier poundages when the amount of work I am doing now is giving mc the growth and definition I want.

Another difference is that my negatives are slower now while my rest periods between sets is shorter. In the past, my negatives were much faster in order to gain the momentum necessary to lift a heavy weight for 6 to 10 reps, so my poundages were heavier. Injuries were more common in training because of this lack of emphasis on the negative.

Now I do more super-setting and get more work done in less time. This means that I have increased the intensity of my workouts and get more pump from a lighter weight by slowing down the negative to make it feel heavier. This slow negative training is a very safe way to train because you have total control over the weight at all times. It is also more conducive for muscle growth. The rule is that your negative should always be slower than your positive.

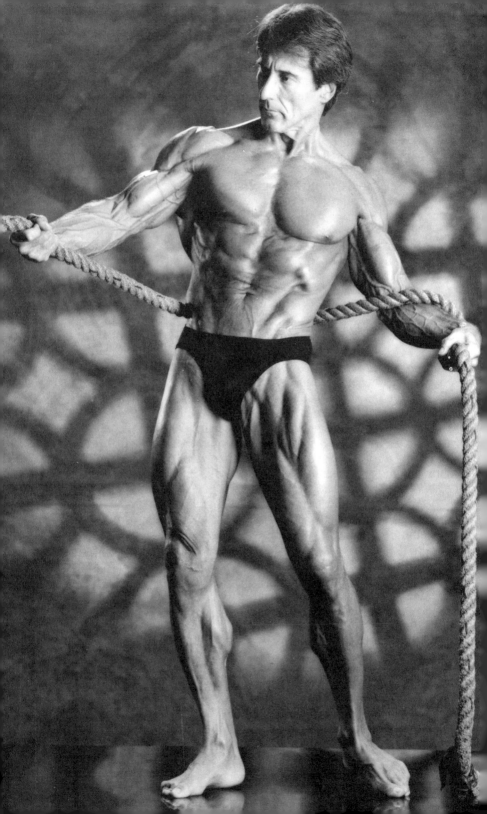

One of my best ever leg workouts took place at my Palm Springs gym on September 11th, 1983, my last year of competition. I awoke at 5:30 am and went for an easy 50 minute bike ride, covering at least 20 km. in the foothils of Palm Springs at dawn. After waiting about 90 minutes for my breakfast of 3 soft boiled eggs, 1/2 tomato, water, and coffee to digest, I started my workout at 8:40 am and trained for 2 hours, doing a total of 34 sets: 15 for calves, and 19 for thighs:

Calves - warmup with one minute of calf stretches
    On Nautilus Multi-Purpose Machine:
    1 Leg Calf Raise - 120/15, 130/15/ 140/15, 150/15, 160/15
    Donkeys - 380/18 drop to 250/10 x 4 sets
    Seated Calf Raise - 100/20, 120/16, 130/15, 140/14, 150/12

Thighs
    Leg Extension - 160/12, 180/11, 200/10, 220/9, 240/7
    Leg Blaster Squat - 120/20, 160/16, 200/12, 220/10
    Lunge on Multi Machine - 90/12, 110/10, 120/10, 130/10
    Leg Curl - 80/12, 90/10, 95/10, 100/8, 105/7, 110/6

Abs - Later in the day I did 950 reps total on abs:
    1 Arm Cable Crunch - 4 sets of 15 reps with 75 pounds
    Seated Twist - 200 non-stop reps

    Hanging Knee up - 6 sets of 25 reps
    Pulley Knee in - 40 pounds: 6 sets of 25 reps

    Incline Leg Raise - 5 sets of 30 reps
    super setted with Crunches - 3 sets of 50 reps
    Hyperextension - 3 sets of 20 reps

Compared to my current leg workouts the above training session uses fewer exercises for calves (3 exercises then, 4 exercises now), as well as for thighs (4 exercises then, 7 exercises now). Since I am doing more exercises, I perform fewer sets, usually averaging 3 sets per exercise.

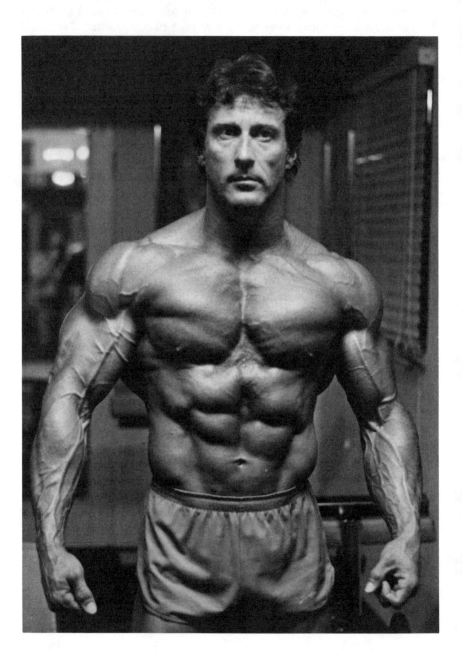

Here is one my best back, biceps, forearms workouts taken from my 1982 training journal that took place in my Palm Springs gym on October 29, 1982, a little over two weeks before the 1982 Olympia in London:

Back

Deadlift from knees up - 235/15, 325/12, 415/10, 485/10, 535/10

Low Cable Row - 180/10, 190/10, 200/10, 210/10, 220/8

1 Arm DB Row - 105/12, 115/11, 125/10

Wide Grip Front Chin - 3 sets of 10 reps super-setted with Close Grip Pulldown - 150/10 - 3 sets

2 Arm DB Row - 50/12, 55/12, 60/10 super-setted with Pulldown Behind Neck - 190/12, 200/10, 180/15

Seated 1 Arm Cable Row - 75/20, 100/16, 110/15, 120/15

Biceps/Forearms

Preacher Cable Curl - 100/15, 110/12, 120/10, 125/9, 130/8

Low Incline DB Curl - 35/12, 40/10, 45/9, 50/8, 50/8

Reverse Preacher Cable Curl - 65/12, 70/10, 70/10, 75/10, 60/8

Barbell Wrist Curl - 90/20, 100/16, 110/12 super-setted w/ Barbell Reverse Curl - 90/10, 100/8, 110/6

Late that evening I did a total of 750 reps of abdominal work.

After expending all this energy training for competition in my late 30's and early 40's, I can appreciate the role that parsimony plays in my workouts as I grow older: Learn to get more benefit out of less exercise. In my 50's, I have been able to stimulate more muscular growth with 2 and 3 sets per exercise than with 4 or 5 sets. Doing more sets would undoubtedly make me overtrained. I don't attempt to use the weights I used 20 years ago because there would be a tremendous risk of injury. Satisfied with the amount of muscle size that I'm maintaining with my current training, my goals now are to keep improving muscular definition, symmetry, and proportion as I grow older.

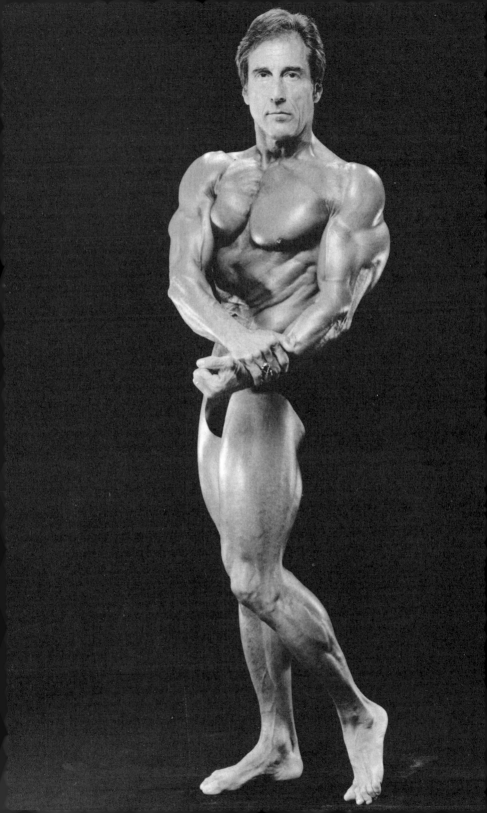

The mature workout is made shorter and more intense with less rest between sets, using moderate weights with slow negatives. The entire workout should take a little more than an hour including abdominal work and aerobics, but not if you are doing 800 reps on abs and 1/2 hour of aerobics. It seems that in order to give the upper body muscle an adequate chance to heal, more rest days between workouts are now necessary. Here is a program I find myself doing when I feel a little more sore and tired than usual:

Day 1 - Back, Biceps, Forearms, Abs, Rowing 500 Meters
Day 2 - Abs, Thighs, Calves, Bike 20 min.
Day 3 - Rest
Day 4 - Chest, Shoulders, Triceps, Abs, Rowing 1000 Meters
Day 5 - Abs, Treadmill 20 minutes.
Day 6 - Rest
Repeat cycle

This 6 day cycle (train 2 days in a row, rest 1 day) gives me 2 days rest between upper body days, allowing my shoulders and elbows plenty of time to release tension, dissipate soreness, and recover.

Opposite page: **FRANK AT AGE 52**

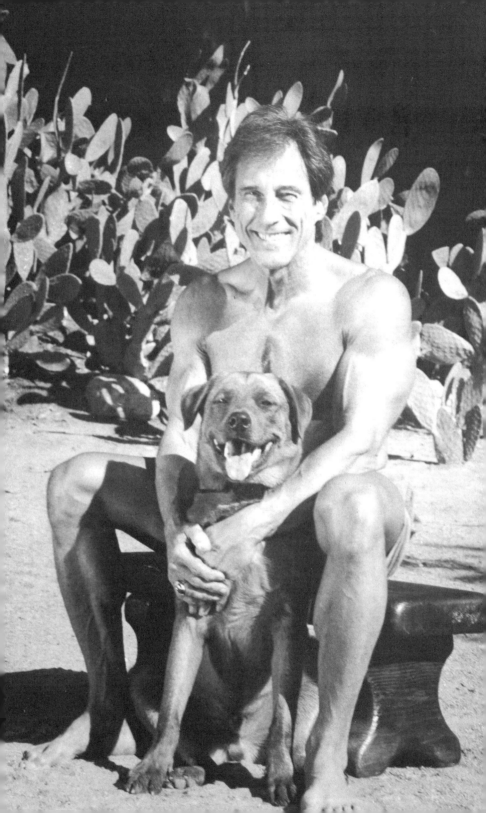

RESOURCES

On one occasion at dusk, a man was feeding his horse with beans from a master's field. The master saw this and called out, "Young man, the beans in that spot are no good. Step further in and you will find better beans for your horse." Hearing this, the man with the horse ran away.

Hisao Inagaki (1)

"Meditation is to find out if there is a field which is not already contaminated by the known."

J. Krishnamurti (2)

The following pages contain information about instruments and equipment that I found useful in my training. These tools are the better beans of the parable, growing in a field unexplored. Venture further into this field and taste progress. I pass this information along to you with advice on how to obtain and use these training tools for mind and body.

Opposite page: **FRANK AND TYLER**

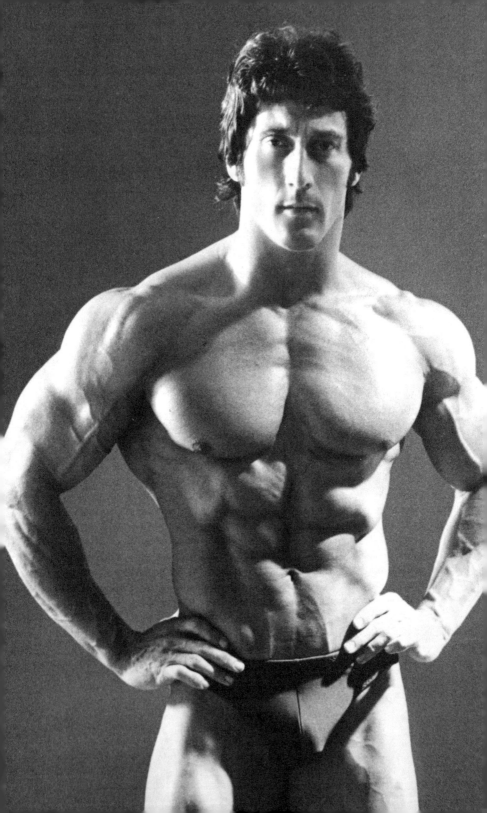

MEDITATION EXERCISE FOR MIND AND BODY

As we grow older, adequate rest and relaxed alertness become more important for muscle building gains and it becomes essential to allow more time to recuperate from hard workouts. If you train less frequently you can train harder. The relation between age and training cycles on pages 166-167 illustrates how less frequent, but more intense intelligent training should increase with age. This is based on my personal experience. In my 20s through age 36, I trained 6 days a week, until I discovered that training three days in a row followed by a rest day helped me feel stronger and train harder. In my late 40s I realized that training 3 days out of 5 (the 5 day cycle) was even better, and now at age 52, I prefer the 6 day cycle to keep my body improving and my enthusiasm peaked. It's the extra recuperation time between workouts that allows the body to repair itself. I maximize these days of rest with meditation: using the electronic mind/body gymnasium I exercise my mind and body with the modalities of light and sound.

I've found the electronic mind/body gym especially helpful in getting past the difficulties encountered in the early stages of meditation, known as the intrusion or distraction stage. During the first several minutes of meditation, the mind wanders a great deal because we are left with nothing to do but concentrate on the meditation object like our breathing or an affirmation which we must remember to keep repeating over and over again. In the beginning, meditation often turns into daydreaming because we forget what we are doing. On the other hand, electronic meditation provides an audio/visual environment conducive to concentration, visualization, energy restoration. I become so absorbed in this new environment that I bypass the boring initial distracting stage of meditation and cut right to the benefits. Electronic meditation leaves me in a profoundly revitalizing cyberspace.

The longer I practice meditation with the electronic mind/body gym while listening to dichotic/beat frequency audio tapes, the more I seem to internalize the meditation process. The light and sound of the meditation seem to download on to the "hard drive" of my mind. In other words, they become part of my memory. Meditation has become easier. Downloaded programs start up when I replicate an element of a regular light/sound session, like the flickering flame of a fireplace, sunlight itself, one of my cats purring, or the sound and sensation of my special vibrating car seat when I'm driving. In learning theory this phenomenon is called stimulus generalization where elements in my everyday environment trigger the calmness I've achieved in meditation.

My attitude seems to improve when my mind is able to relax at will. Edmund Jacobson, the father of Progressive Relaxation concluded that all thoughts are accompanied by skeletal muscle activity, even though it may be at a very low level. Conversely, he also found that thought processes diminished and eventually disappeared as the skeletal muscles relaxed. Relax your skeletal muscles and you clear your mind, improve concentration and performance, and ease nervous tension. Distracting or disturbing thoughts lose their potency if the muscles are completely relaxed. In Jacobson's words, "It might be naive to say that we think with our muscles, but it would be inaccurate to say that we think without them." (3)

I've learned that the best thing a bodybuilder can do to help regain energy is to practice meditation. I make it my goal to have an extended meditation session several hours after my workout. Intensive workouts increase your need for energy restoration.

THE RHYTHM METHOD

Rhythm means regularity of movement, movement in time to a beat. Rhythm is measured by beat frequency. If a movement has a beat frequency of 1 hz. this means the movement ocurs one time each second; 2 hz. means the movement occurs two times each second, etc. Beat frequency tells us the rate at which rhythm is occurring. To get the best pump during a set your reps should have a beat frequency: I do one rep every four seconds to build size, and one rep every two seconds for high rep exercises like abdominals. I've recorded audio tapes which synchronize and slow the negative of each rep to the rhythmic tone coming into my headphones.

I've also produced audio tapes for stationary bicycling, walking on treadmill, stairclimber, and rowing which contain beat frequencies. The optimum cycling cadence is 90 revolutions per minute which equals 1.5 hz. or 1 and 1/2 revolutions each second. Rowing is whatever rate you are comfortable with for an easy row (about 25 strokes per minute or 0.4 hz. for me) or a hard competitive row (about 30 strokes a minute or 0.5 hz). Walking cadence depends on how fast you want to walk. I average 3 miles per hour with my 16 inch stride which makes my beat frequency for waking 3.3 hz., a low theta wave frequency near the delta borderline associated with deep rest.

What is interesting to me is that the beat frequencies of working out aerobically as well as anaerobically with weights are in the lowest brainwave frequency range: Delta waves, the brainwaves of deep sleep where growth hormone is released by the anterior pituitary. Is it possible that the deep delta wave frequency of rhythmic repetitions with slow negatives is related to the GH release associated with doing your sets in a weight-training workout at maximum intensity?

THE ULTIMATE BENEFITS OF MEDITATION

Aside from all the physcial and psychological benefits of meditation are transpersonal effects which have the potential to effect large numbers of people. Remarkable findings known as TM Social Field Effects (4) show when one percent of the individuals in a community of 10,000 to 50,000 population practiced TM, there was a significant drop in the crime rate.

Sophisticated research has replicated these results and further show evidence of a significant 8.2% decrease in crime in the experimental cities practicing TM, while at the same time there was an increase of 8.3% in the matched control cities. This means a difference of 16.5% in the crime rates of cities with one percent of its people meditating and cities without this critical population of meditators. Based on the outcome of these studies, as more and more people become skilled in meditation techniques and continue to practice, crime may eventually disappear and world peace will prevail!

The scientific explanation for TM Social Field Effects postulates when a critical mass is attained, a pervading influence encourages a more harmonious organization among all group members (5). Itzak Bentov (6) explains:

> Techniques for extending this harmonious resonant state have been known for thousands of years. These are the different meditative techniques...The resonant state will naturally apply to the whole body. The skeleton and all the inner organs will move coherently at about 7 cycles per second...When a charged body is vibrating, it is coupled to the electrostatic field of the planet. This vibration causes a regular repetitive signal or wave to propagate within this field. This signal will naturally have the tendency to entrain any body vibrating at frequencies close to it. In other words, if there are other people in the vicinity or anywhere on the globe who are meditating and approaching

this resonant frequency (7 hz.) they will be pushed along and locked into that frequency...Thus the more bodies that are locked in, the stronger the signal becomes...(and) It pleases the planet no end to have such an accompaniment to its tune. (pp. 42-44)

THE BRAINWARE 200 MIND/BODY GYMNASIUM

A person who practices mind/body exercise can improve mental concentration and relax at will, stay calm in stressful situations, and revitalize himself or herself as needed. Consider these facts: Disciplined meditators exhibit biological ages up to 12 years younger than their chronological ages. Engineers at Seiko Instruments in Japan successfully achieved 30% more patents as a result of Alpha Brainwave Training. One particular study showed meditative visualization built strength far better than psyching up. Yes, meditation raises both physical and mental performance (7).

The *Brainware 200* (or *B-200*) is a piece of electronic equipment designed specifically to maximize mind/body meditation exercises. The *B-200* uses a micro-processor and advanced electronics to program the complex multi-layered characteristics of light and sound, resulting in an environment most conducive to mind/body exercises. Its unique finger temperature sensor gauges your mastery of your mind/body connection, so you can measure your progress.

This kind of technology opens the door to greater mind/body excellence for many people. It is probably the most important invention since modern day weight training equipment. In the past people who were dedicated to getting the most out of their lives through achieving excellence through training, were limited to physical exercise only. The potential of the mind had been largely ignored. Now with this new technology, we can train our mind as well as our body to achieve mind/body excellence. This wholistic approach not only brings bodybuilding and sports performance to a new level, but also raises mental and cognitive performance to new heights.

Looking into the future, I realize that bodybuilding will grow into mind/bodybuilding and adopt the pursuit of excellence as defined in the new mind/body paradigm. Just as in the Golden Age of Greece (8) where:

314

The people met in one grand intellectual, social, artistic, and gymnastic assembly, which had great use in fostering a common national pride, a sound physical training, intellectual vigor and emulation, and a healthy desire for success in every kind of competition, where the reward consisted cheifly in the high opinions won from fellow men.

To learn more about mind/body exercise and the Brainware 200 mind/body gymnasium, write to Cognitech Corporation, 124 Mt. Auburn St., University Place, Harvard Square, Cambridge, MA 02138 or call 800-844-6527.

CAUTION: People who have epilepsy, or any abnormal neurological condition should not use the *Brainware 200.*

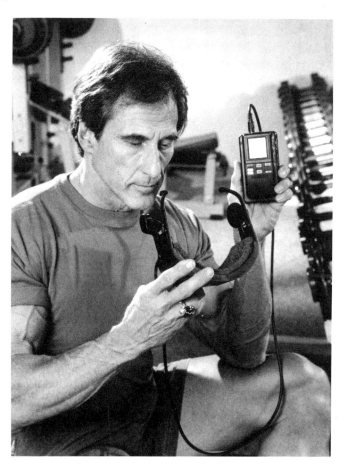

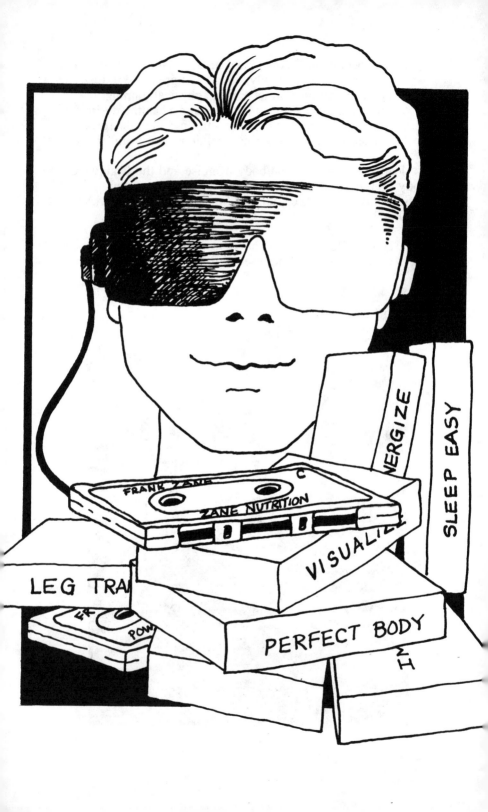

DICHOTIC AUDIO TAPES

These cassettes are recorded using the dichotic technique where you listen to two stories at the same time, one in each ear through headphones. You sometimes pay attention to the left ear message, the right ear message, both messages, or neither of the messages. Where and how you pay attention doesn't matter because dichotics relies on the conscious mind's natural tendency to wander and not pay attention. Listening dichotically, you spontaneously let go of the effort of paying attention, relax, and absorb positive suggestions. Messages and affirmations seem to register in memory unconsciously and can later help to improve your concentration and workout performance.

Listening to the sounds recorded on these high quality chrome audio cassettes is the easiest, most cost effective way to experience the meditative state. All you need is your cassette player and headphones and these tapes to soothe you into a pleasant euphoric state and give you suggestions to motivate your training and improve the quality of your relaxation and performance. Since the thoughts you are thinking right now dictate your present mood, these dichotic audio tapes can improve your attitude and enhance goal directed behaviors. These audio tapes can also increase the effectiveness of your light/sound meditation sessions with the electronic mind gym.

THE BEAT FREQUENCY TAPES #s 12, 13, 15, 16, 17, 18, & 20 contain primordial sounds like ocean waves, nature sounds, chords, and tones of varying pitch and binaural beat frequencies intended to enhance different behavioral effects. Although these tapes do not contain messages or suggestions, we have found the modulated beat frequencies to be powerful in producing the desired result.

Here is a list and description of the Dichotic & Beat Frequency audio cassettes we've created:

TAPE 1 - **THE BLUEPRINT** on side 1 is for visualization and goal setting, and **THE MAGIC PUMP** on side 2 is for workout motivation and performance, and getting psyched-up for competition.

TAPE 2 - **THE POWER CELL** on side 1 helps you relax and improve concentration, and **THE DREAM RECOVERY** on side 2 uses dichotics for recuperating after hard workouts with deep relaxation.

TAPE 3 - **IMAGINE YOURSELF THINNER** on side 1 Christine uses a filmstrip visualization technique to motivate fat loss, and **INTENSIFY AEROBICS** on side 2 she helps you stay with your stationary aerobic exercise longer and burn more calories.

TAPE 4 - **HEALTHY WEIGHT LOSS** on side 1 Christine motivates appetite control and correct eating, and **EMERGE FROM YOUR SHELL** on side two she gives powerful dichotic suggestions for improving self-esteem and confidence as you improve your looks.

TAPE 5 - **TRAIN UPPER BODY** on side 1 Frank gets you psyched up for your upper body workout, while **LEG TRAIN** on side 2 motivates you to train harder in your leg workout.

TAPE 6 - **THE BICYCLE RACE** on side 1 is the tape Frank used for his Master's thesis in psychology, *The Effect of Dichotic Listening on Aerobic Performance.* This tape helped people ride a stationary bike longer and burn more calories. Side 2, **THE WALK** is designed to motivate you to walk longer while on your treadmill.

TAPE 7 - **CLIMB** on side 1 gives you positive suggestions and motivation to workout longer on your stairclimber and **ROW**, side 2 coordinates your rowing cadence to 25 strokes per minute and lets you relax and row longer on your rowing machine.

TAPE 8 - **POSITIVE ATTITUDE** is all about relaxing and re-programming negative self talk with positive affirmations. Since most of our self talk is negative, this tape may be a valuable tool for self improvement when used on a regular basis.

TAPE 9 - **SLEEP EASY** is a dichotic body visualization which you can listen to while in bed before you fall asleep. Side 2 soothes you with delta wave binaural beat frequencies.

TAPE 10 - **ZANE NUTRITION** employs peripheral affirmations that motivate you to eat correctly by choosing the best foods for fat loss, energy expenditure, and building lean muscle mass.

TAPE 11 - **PERFECT BODY** uses a relaxing time/space-line visualization designed to motivate you to adopt the necesary behaviors to improve your body.

TAPE 12 - **SOOTHING SOUNDS** lets you relax to descending binaural beat frequencies and dichotic ocean waves. Side 1 contains beta through alpha frequencies which we like for relaxed concentration. Side 2 uses high theta to low delta for use before bed.

TAPE 13 - **MIND MELODY** contains beat frequencies embedded in beautifully relaxing music to lull you into an ecstatic mood.

TAPE 14 - **POWER PHRASE** on side 1 uses affirmations from *Fabulously Fit Forever* to replace negative internal dialog & change negative attitudes. Side 2, **GAIN WITHOUT PAIN** uses dichotics to help change attitudes toward hard training and overcome soreness.

TAPE 15 - **ENERGIZE** on side 1 is perfect for listening to upon awakening in the morning, with binaural beat frequencies and modulated ocean waves from delta up to Schumann Resonance Frequency of 7.83 hz. Side 2 takes you from 7.83 hz up to high beta waves to get focused before your workouts.

TAPE 16 - **VISUALIZE** is a mixture of surf, musical chords, and oscillating binaural beat frequencies which sweep down so you can relax -- intended to help you evoke mental imagery while you meditate and visualize.

THE WORKOUT TAPES 17 AND 18 are designed to pace you through each set of your workout by helping you synchronize the speed of the negative or eccentric phase of each of your repetitions. You learn to slow down and control your negative and do your reps with perfect rhythm. To achieve this effect, Frank has produced these unique recordings for listening to with headphones while you work out. Using beat frequencies in the low delta wave range, you synchronize your body movements involved in each exercise to the beat.

TAPE 17 - **MAXIMIZE MUSCLE SIZE** - Gain muscle size and strength by slowing your negative down to 0.29 hz. This means you do approximately 1 rep every 4 seconds. You should use a lighter weight at first until you connect with the right speed and rhythm, then increase the weight on your second and third sets. Frank especially likes to use this tape for working the bigger muscle groups like thighs, chest, and back. You focus into a groove where you forget about how many reps you've done and just keep going for an ultimate burn!

TAPE 18 - **DEFINITELY DEFINITION** - Lose bodyfat and increase muscular definition by doing more reps with a faster negative. Frank uses a delta beat frequency of 0.5 seconds (one rep every two seconds), and mixes in high energy beta waves to keep you pumping hard throughout your entire workout. Great for faster higher rep movements like abdominal, forearm and calf work. Use both tapes to really shock your muscles!

TAPE 19 - **DICHOTIC FABULOUSLY FIT FOREVER** - Frank narrates passages from *Fabulously Fit Forever* and mixes them into one dichotic tape that you can listen to with headphones with your left ear only, or only with your right ear for information, or you can listen with both ears simultaneously to relax and learn. 2 tapes in one!

TAPE 20 - **ULTIMATE GH SOUNDS** is a complex mix of delta wave binaural beat frequencies of 0.29 hz, 1.0 hz, and 1.5 hz to help you relax and grow. An incredibly mesmerizing sound!

TAPE 21 - **DICHOTIC DEEP RELAXATION**, side 1 is great for relaxing with during the day or night, **DREAM BODY VISUALIZATION** side 2 enhances the mental imagery foundation for the future body of your dreams.

TAPES 22, 23, 24, 25, 26, & 27 are designed to **quickly** elicit energized concentration, relaxed alertness, and deep states of rest. These tapes contain binaural beat frequencies, nature sounds, and chords of different pitch which sweep up, down, or hover within a certain desired range. Frank uses powerful techniques such as phase shifting where voice and tones travel from ear to ear, metaphors, and embedded suggestions to help you achieve your desired mood and frame of mind as quickly as 10 to 15 minutes. Or if you wish to deepen the desired effect, you can listen for the entire 25 minutes on each side.

TAPE 22 - **UNWIND** mixes organ chords and descending beat frequencies with peripheral affirmations conducive to deep relaxation. Perfect for using after a stressful day at work or before bed.

TAPE 23 - **MEDITATE** uses frequencies descending into the alpha range which produce a pleasant singing wave. It provides instruction which helps you bring your attention back to focusing on your breathing.

TAPE 24 - **PEAK PERFORMANCE** combines resonating cello chords and alpha beat frequencies with affirmations for doing your very best in the task at hand. Great before workouts or sports competition.

TAPE 25 - **FOCUS** mixes two ascending frequencies from theta up to high alpha with suggestions intended to create a relaxed alertness and improve concentration before workouts or sports competition.

TAPE 26 - **LEARN** side 1 contains alpha beat frequencies and nature sounds with suggestion for learning to use before studying. Side 2 contains descending theta wave frequencies with suggestions for absorbing material into memory after you've studied (Side 2 is ideal to use before bed).

TAPE 27 - **SLEEP SOUND** uses beat frequencies descending into the delta range with suggestions for drowsiness. Wonderful to use as a prelude to sleep or before taking a nap.

EACH UNIQUE AUDIO TAPE IS **$14.95 + $2** POSTAGE.
BUY 3 TAPES AND GET 1 FREE! **$44.85 + $3** POSTAGE.
ANY 10 TAPES OF YOUR CHOICE **$110** POSTPAID.
SAVE $100! ALL 27 AUDIO TAPES **$269** POSTPAID.

THE PERFECT HOME GYM

Many people prefer training in a home gym for at least some of their workouts because of its many advantages. A well equipped home gym provides a place to train whenever you want without any of the distractions of a commercial gym. It is more convenient, more cost effective in the long run, and can save a lot of time for people with busy schedules. Be sure to buy the very best equipment for your home gym. You will get great workouts and it will last a long long time. If you buy junk -- and there is a lot of it out there -- you have a hard time giving it away.

I have built 6 home gyms during my 38 year training career. As I learned and saved my money, each suceeding gym got better and better. My first home gym, which I built in my basement at age 15, consisted of a flat bench, barbell, squat rack, and adjustable dumbells. My next two gyms were in schools where I taught. They had lots of free weights plus a lat machine and and calf machine. Next came my home gym in Florida in 1968 which had a combination Smith machine/lat machine, fixed dumbbells from 10's to 65's, parallel dip bars, and an Olympic bar and plates.

After moving to Southern California in 1969, I trained at the original Gold's Gym up until it closed in 1976, then at World Gym and Gold's Gym in Venice until I moved to Palm Springs in 1985. My gym at Zane Haven was the biggest and best equipped gym to date with over 750 square feet of floor space and fixed dumb bells up to 100 lbs, Nautilus Leg Extension, leg curl, and multi-purpose machine, and combination power rack/pulldown/low cable row, cable crossover machine, and the prototype for the Leg Blaster.

In 1988 we moved to our current location and my gym is the best ever, with over 1100 square feet of floor space filled with my favorite machines and free weights. Over the years I have had the opportunity to attend many weight-training equipment trade shows and work out on all types of apparatus to determine what is the very best. Here is the equipment I recommend for your home gym:

THE ALL NEW LEG BLASTER

Yes, the squat is the best exercise for developing the thighs. But it is hard on the knees and lower back, can enlarge the buttocks and waistline, and it's uncomfortable to hold the barbell in position on the shoulders. Now you can develop your legs without the discomfort of barbell squats. The Leg Blaster gives you the benefit of all versions of squatting just by changing your foot position. Since your hands are free you don't have to hold on to the weight. Just hold the balance bar to make sure you are in perfect position.

Its two main parts, the harness and the rack, make up the complete unit and are not sold seperately. The harness is handsomely styled and features an all new stabilizing latch for easy connection to the rack, which prevents tipping while loading. Comfortably padded at the shoulder and ribcage contact points, its plateholders (choose regular or Olympic size) will easily accommodate all size barbell plates. The rack is specially designed to hold the harness while you load it. It has a beautiful powder coated finish and is entirely free standing, provides rear plate storage, and requires no bolting to the floor. Its heavy duty single post construction assembles in minutes and will fit into the most crowded gym.

The All New Leg Blaster will replace the squat rack and even the leg press machine where space is a premium. It is a real bargain at **$499** + UPS. (Price reduced $200 from former model)

FRANK'S NEW LEG BLASTER VIDEO

Learn Frank's squatting secrets and how to get fantastic calves!....only **$9.95 + $3** shipping or **FREE** WITH LEG BLASTER PURCHASE!

THE BACK REVOLUTION is the best way I found to give traction to the lower back and it is a great hyperextension bench as well. Many people come up too far on the hyperextension exercise, compressing the lower back. The Back Revolution emphasis the stretch portion of this exercise and minimizes the lower back compression produced by many convention hyperextension benches and lower back machines. This movement is essential for people with low back problems. It is well worth the cost of **$399** plus UPS.

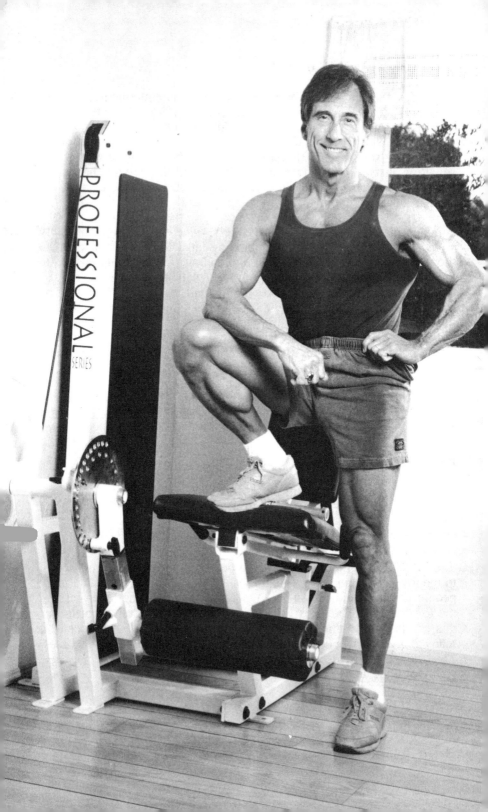

PRO COMBO LEG EXTENSION/CURL MACHINE - Without a doubt, this the finest combination unit available. Equipped with a 150 or 200 pound weight stack, it is a perfect piece for the home gym since it works the entire quadriceps with leg extension, and hamstrings with leg curl. It is only $1895 plus freight.

PRO HOME LAT MACHINE is a very well made lat pulldown/low cable row with a 150 or 200 pound weight stack which is ideal for home use. It is $1695 plus freight.

PRO ADJUSTABLE FLAT/INCLINE BENCH is a sturdy, quick adjusting bench for $295.

AFS DUMB BELLS are the industry standard (average cost is about $2 a pound) and the chromed BEAUTY BELLS (10 pairs 2/5 to 25 pounds in 2.5 pound jumps) have nicely contoured handles, fit into a very compact rack and are favorites of personal trainers.

PREFERENCE HRT 2000 SEMI-RECUMBENT STATIONARY BICYCLE is a lifesaver that has replaced upright stationary cycling for me which can be used anywhere because it requires no plug in. This is a heavy smooth comfortable bike with programs and heart rate monitor, but I just use it manually. I begin to pedal, gradually increase the resistance into the 60 to 100 watt range at 80 to 100 cadence, and ride for 15 to 30 minutes. Price is $1995 plus freight.

YOU CAN ORDER ANY OF THE ABOVE EQUIPMENT BY CONTACTING ME AT 800-323-7537 OR 619-323-7486 IN CALIFORNIA, OR FAX ME AT 619-323-2888.

VALEO WEIGHT LIFTING BELT - Nowadays, I wear the Valeo Belt for virtually all exercises except abdominal work and leg curls. The Valeo Belt is best because of its cloth form fitting construction, its quick velcro fastener, and its light weight and flexibility. This belt is a must to wear during your workout if you have a sore back. For info call Valeo at 800-634-2704.

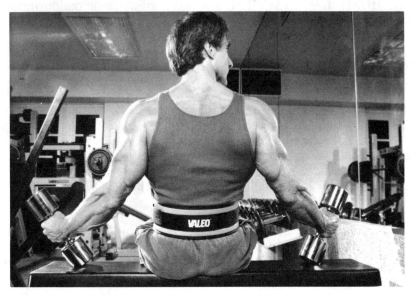

PRECOR 9.4 E/L TREADMILL - I especially like the courses 9 and 10 varied from 2 degrees decline up to 12 degrees incline, as well as the manual mode. This gives me a great workout for the fron and back of my legs. This is a nice unit for the home and costs $3400. Although designed for health clubs, Precor's top of the line treadmill, the C-964 is a superb machine for home use as well and runs in the $5000 range. Call 206-486-9292 to locate the Precor dealer nearest you.

CONCEPT II ROWING ERGOMETER MODEL C is a bigger more solid version of Model B (I've owned a Model B for over 8 years). It is a bargain at $700 and one of the finest aerobic machine that works the whole body. The nice thing about rowing is that 5 minutes a day will go a long way in strengthening the lower back and tightening up the waistline. The legs get worked too along with all the muscles of the back, delts, biceps, triceps, and forearms. To order call 800-245-5676.

I can help you obtain **MY FAVORITE FOOD SUPPLEMENTS**:

ENZYMATIC THERAPY **LIVER EXTRACT** is five times as strong as desiccated liver and 20 times a concentrated as calves liver. I feel more strength and energy when I use take 3 or 4 capsules with each meal. Each pure concentrated cold processed liquid capsule contains 550 mg. of 20 to 1 concentrated liver extract plus 100 mcg. of vitamin B-12 and NO FATS OR CHOLESTEROL.

90 capsules...........$20   180 capsules...........$35

ENZYMATIC THERAPY **STEROPLEX** is a blend of essential fatty acids from germ oil concentrates, lecithin, saw palmetto berry oil, vitamins and minerals to supplement the body's own natural steroid production related to strength and sexual function. This a great way to add the right kind of fats to the diet. I take 1 or 2 capsules with meals.

60 capsules............$15   120 capsules.............$25

ENZYMATIC THERAPY **MEGA-ZYME** DIGESTIVE ENZYMES are 10 times stronger than regular pancreatin and contain all the enzymes necessary to assist in digestion of protein, carbohydrate, and fat. Christine and I take 2 or 3 soft tablets with each meal.

100 tablets............$20   200 tablets...............$35

AMINO MULTI PACS are a convenient way to get encapsulated free form amino acids, vitamins, and minerals. Each packet contains 3 amino acid capsules, 2 multi-vitamin-mineral capsules, and 1 high potency B complex capsule, and provides 2100 mg. of pharmaceutical grade FREE FORM AMINO ACIDS of the highest purity: L-Lysine, Glycine, L-Leucine, L-Methionine, L-Arginine, L-Valine, L-Phenylalanine, L-Isoleucine, L-Histidine, L-Threonine, L-Tyrosine, L-Glutamic Acid. VITAMINS: A - 8000 i.u., C - 100 mg, B-1 - 65 mg., B-2 - 45 mg., Niacin - 20 mg., Niacinamide - 75 mg., B-12 - 420 mcg., Folic Acid - 360 mcg., Biotin - 420 mcg., PABA - 90 mg., Vitamin E - 120 i.u., Choline Bitartrate - 125 mg., Inositol - 50 mg., and MINERALS: Calcium - 80 mg., Magnesium - 50 mg., Potassium - 39 mg., Manganese - 6 mg., Zinc - 12 mg., Copper 60 mcg., Selenium - 40 mcg., Molybdenum - 60 mcg., Chromium - 60 mcg., Iron - 7.2 mg., Iodine - 30 mcg. I feel more energy and strength when I take one packet right before each meal.

AMINO STRESS PACS are designed to assist in the metabolic management of acute and chronic stress, as well as for compromised nutritional function. This is a broad spectrum multiple amino acid formula containing 18 L-crystalline amino acids including the 9 essentials: L-Lysine, L-Arginine, L-Isoleucine, L-Leucine, L-Alanine, L-Threonine, L-Histidine, L-Cystine, L-Methionine, L-Glutamine, L-Tyrosine, L-Aspartic Acid, L-Valine, L-Glutamic Acid, L-Phenylalanine, Glycine, L-Serine, L-Cysteine. This formula is a rich source of the neuro-transmitter precursors and sulfur amino acids. These pharmaceutical high grade amino acids are contained in two capsules and supply 260 mg. of nitrogen. Due to the participation of vitamins and minerals in amino acid metabolism and tissue maintenance, a high potency vitamin-mineral capsule is included in the packet, along with a pyridoxal 5` phosphate tablet designed to release in the small intestine. This is the active form of Vitamin B-6 which participates in the synthesis of non-essential amino acids and overall amino acid transport and conversion in the body, and is suppested as having a minimizing effect on certain drug/nutrient interactions. We find this product great to balance the stress of strict dieting when one packet is taken before meals. Christine takes one packet before each meal and I take one packet before bed since I feel a relaxing effect from it.

PRICES OF AMINO MULTI PACS OR AMINO STRESS PACS:

60 Packets ...**$65** (+ $3 postage), 120 packets ...**$125** includes postage.

METAFORM Technically Advanced Nutrition Packets from Fitness Systems are the handiest, tastiest, and most nutritious meal replacement I've ever found. They are better than Met-Rx! I mix 2 packets for breakfast and the same for dinner (see my recipe on page 185) and include a quick shake in my blender which I sip after my workout. Each packet provides 37 grams of protein, 24 grams of carbs, 2 grams of fat, and only 200 mg of sodium. I use both the original and the chocolate flavors, add a teaspoon of psyllium and fruit and make the perfect delicious meal that satisfies my appetite for desserts! Cost is $2.50 per serving packet. METAFORM is distributed by Great American Nutrition and is available at GNC stores.

BOOKS BY FRANK AND CHRISTINE

ZANE NUTRITION

Now at last for this generation of athletic Americans comes the total nutrition book. Whether you practice weight training, do aerobics, run, play tennis, *Zane Nutrition* is a lifetime regimen for people who exercise as well as for serious athletes. This is not a book about dieting; it is a book about eating correctly for optimum fitness and improved personal appearance, and offers complete information on:

How your body uses protein, carbs, fats, vitamins and minerals
What you should and should not eat
How to lose, gain, and maintain bodyweight
How to buy, prepare, & serve food for most nutritional benefit
When and how to use food supplements
How to prepare complete menus and many wonderful recipes
A 21 Day Eating Plan and much more

Zane Nutrition is based upon the author's own personal experience as professional weight trainers and owners of The Zane Experience. Their common sense approach eliminates the ups and downs of fanatical dieting. You eat a wide variety of delicious nutritious foods that will give you energy and provide for growth and repair of muscles, internal organs, bones, skin and hair. *Zane Nutrition* is a crucial ingredient that every active person needs in order to stay in shape and maintain a life of health and vigor. 256 pages **$16.95** postpd.

THE COOKBOOK COMPANION TO ZANE NUTRITION

Even more delicious easy to prepare low-fat recipes in addition to *ZANE NUTRITION*. We prefer meals created with a minimum of ingredients and cooking time. The *COOKBOOK* contains a wide variety of appetizing and nutritious dishes that are both fast and easy to prepare: salads, soups, cereals, pasta, grains, vegetables, fish, meats, poultry, eggs, herbs and spices, fruit drinks, and many tasty desserts. The *COOKBOOK* teaches you to use your favorite foods, herbs, and spices and combine them to create meals that are uniquely yours. Its spiral bound 8 & 1/2 by 11 inch format will stay open to the page you want so you can follow instructions easily. There's room for notes and helpful hints that enable you to cook dishes your friends will envy. Beautifully illustrated by Christine, the *COOKBOOK* will keep you dining in style while staying in great shape. **$16.95** postpaid

BUY THE COOKBOOK & ZANE NUTRITION .. $25 POSTPAID

I WILL HELP YOU BUILD YOUR HOME GYM

Please feel free to call me and I will help you order the equipment you want. Contact me to order the following items: Dichotic and Beat Frequency Audio Tapes, The New Leg Blaster, The Back Revolution, AFS Dumb Bells, Pro Leg Extension/Leg Curl Machine, Pro Lat Machine, Pro Adjustable Bench, and Preference HRT Semi-Recumbent Bike. Cognitech's Brainware 200, Precor Treadmills, Valeo Lifting Belts, and Concept II Rowing Ergometers can be contacted directly. I will be happy to personally demonstrate this equipment when you come to Palm Srpings for a private Zane Experience Seminar.

THE ZANE EXPERIENCE is the name of my private one-to-one training seminars. You will train with me personally in my private gym in Palm Springs. Fully equipped with the very best exercise machines, free weights, and *Brainware 200* Mind/Body Training Systems, my training facility is totally unique and one of the world's finest. I will design a training program just for you and show you everything you need to get in the best shape of your life.

We'll arrange three private 2 & 1/2 hour sessions over three days to best fit your schedule. I will personally analyze your diet and show you how to eat correctly and use food supplements to maximize your potential. And you'll experience deep relaxation and enhance your training motivation in my mind gym with dichotic audio tapes and the *Brainware 200*. Your private Zane Experience will save you years of trial and error in your training. You'll learn precise techniques for over 60 exercises, stretches, and training shortcuts that will speed your progress. Save paying a personal trainer by returning in the future as often as you like to upgrade your program and stay motivated.

Our training sessions will be completely private or you can bring a friend and I will work with both of you at the same time. You pay only **$475** each when you come with a friend or **$575** when you come alone. I can help you arrange hotel accommodations, recommend the best restaurants, and help you plan your Palm Springs vacation. If your time is limited we'll do a 2 & 1/2 hour private session and start you on a complete training and nutritional program for **$195**.

Interested in training under my direct supervision on a regular basis? One hour individual workouts are **$125** a session or **$175** for 2 people training together. Get started right now by calling me at 619-323-7486 to arrange a time for your Zane Experience. Fill out the Resistration Form and mail it along with full payment or fax it (619-323-2888) to us with your Visa, MasterCard, Discover, or American Express number and expiration date. I look forward to train with you!

REGISTRATION FORM

Dear Frank,

Enclosed is $_____ in full payment for my private Zane Experience on the dates of _____. I understand that all of my sessions will be entirely with you personally.

NAME_____AGE_____SEX____

STREET_____

CITY_____STATE_____ZIP_____

PHONE_____HEIGHT_____WEIGHT_____

OCCUPATION_____PRIOR WT. TRAINING_____YRS.

MY GOALS ARE:

_____

_____

_____

_____

_____

DO YOU HAVE ANY SERIOUS INJURIES OR DISABILITIES?___

IF YES, PLEASE ATTACH A NOTE FROM A MEDICAL DOCTOR PERMITTING YOU TO DO OUR PROGRAM.

I HOLD FRANK ZANE FREE FROM ALL LIABILITY AND FULLY UNDERSTAND THAT I PARTICIPATE IN THE ACTIVITIES AT ZANE EXPERIENCE AT MY OWN RISK AND THAT NO REFUND IS GIVEN.

SIGNED_____DATE_____

USE THIS HANDY ORDER FORM

DEAR FRANK,

PLEASE SEND ME THE FOLLOWING PRODUCTS. I UNDERSTAND THAT SOME WILL BE SENT DIRECTLY FROM YOU WHILE OTHERS (SUCH AS WEIGHT TRAINING EQUIPMENT) WILL BE SHIPPED DIRECTLY FROM THE MANUFACTURER. I HAVE CIRCLED THE ITEMS I WANT:

Fabulously Fit Forever Expanded Book $19.95 + $3 postage
Zane Nutrition Book $13.95 + $3
Cookbook Companion to Zane Nutrition $13.95 + $3
Zane Nutrition + Cookbook $25 postpaid
Amino Multi Pacs 60 pacs $65 + $3, 120 pacs $125 postpaid
Amino Stress Pacs 60 pacs $65 + $3, 120 pacs $125 postpaid
Liver Extract 90 caps $20, 180 caps $35 + $3
Steroplex 60 caps $20, 120 caps $25 + $3
Megazyme Digestive Enzymes 100 tabs $20, 200 tabs $35 + $3
Audio Tapes $14.95 each + $2 postage
Buy 3 tapes, get one free $44.85 + $3
Any 10 tapes $110 postpaid
All 27 tapes $269 postpaid
The All New Leg Blaster $499 + UPS
The New Leg Blaster Video $12.95 postpaid
The Back Revolution $399 + UPS
AFS Dumb Bells - Call for quotes
Preference HRT Recumbent Stationary Bike $1995 + freight
Pro Leg Extension/Leg Curl $1895 + freight
Pro Lat Machine $1695 + freight
Pro Adjustable Bench $295 + freight

TOTAL ORDER_____ + 7.75% tax in CA. + shipping = _____

To order by Visa, MasterCard, Discover, or American Express, call 1-800-323-7537 or 619-323-7486 in CA., or fax 1-619-323-2888. Or you can send us a money order (gets faster service than a personal check) to Zane Experience, PO Box 2031, Palm Springs, CA 92263.

Opposite page: **FRANK AT 52**

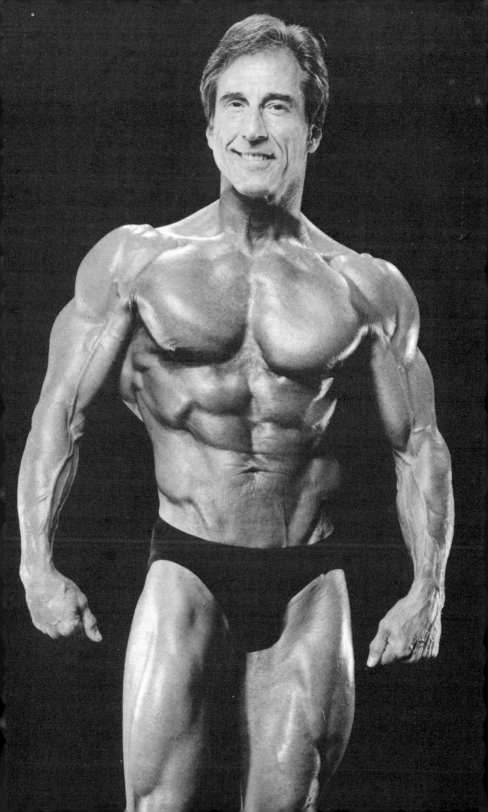

REFERENCES TO RECOURCES SECTION

1. Inagaki, H. (1992). *Shinran and Jodoshinshu.* IABC Pamphlet Series.

2. Krishnamurti, J. (1979). *Meditations.* New York: Harper & Row, Page 26.

3. Neuro-Technology Research Corporation (1994). *Mind Machine Buyers Guide.* Cambridge, Ma.

4. Borland, C., & Landrith, G., (1977). Improved quality of city life through the Transcendental Meditaiton program: Decreased crime rate. In Orme-Johnson & Farrow (Eds.), *Scientific research on the Transcendental Meditaiton Program: Collected papers* (Vol. 1, 2nd Ed., pp. 639-648). Livingston Manor, NY: Maharishi European Research University Press.

5. Lichstein, K.L. (1988). *Clinical Relaxation Strategies.* New York: John Wiley & sons, P. 303.

6. Bentov, I. (1988). *Stalking the Wild Pendulum.* Rochester, Vt.: Destiny Books, pp. 42-44.

7. Cognitech Corporation. (1995). *The Brainware 200 Companion User's Manual.* Cambridge, Ma.: University Place, 124 Mount Auburn St., Suite 200, Harvard Square, Cambridge, Ma. 02138.

8. Sanderson, E., Lamberton, J.P., McGovern, J., & Leigh, O. (1901). *Six Thousand Years of History.* Volume 1. Chicago: Dumont. p. 156.